Praise for *But You Look So Normal: Lost and Found in a Hearing World*

"Marseille's memoir is a beautifully told, nostalgic portrayal of a 1950s childhood with a severe hearing loss. Born at a time when hearing aids were crude amplifiers, Claudia had to deal with loneliness at school, social gatherings, and professional demands. She finally learned to tell others about her hearing loss and find meaning in a loving marriage and a successful career as a painter. Hers is an evocative story of resilience, and her challenges will resonate with anyone who has experienced hearing loss."

—Katherine Bouton, president of the Hearing Loss
Association of America, NYC Chapter, and author of
Shouting Won't Help and *Smart Hearing*

"Claudia boldly shares with us a heartwarming story, unveiling the challenges of a significant and isolating disability and heartbreaking insights into complicated relationships. Her persistence to overcome these obstacles and 'fit in' help us grow to deeply appreciate her numerous natural talents, bravery, beauty, all within the threads of a grounded and humble woman—who may not fully appreciate her incredible brilliance."

—Jill Ellis, MEd, cofounder of Center for Early intervention on Deafness

"Marseille's skilled, down-to-earth, deeply moving, and bravely intimate storytelling is a captivating look at the profound lifelong impacts of growing up and finding one's way as an adult with a severe hearing loss in a hearing world. Yet, while hearing loss is central to her story, it is also about the many experiences that has created the tapestry of a life rich with complex relationships, passionate artistic talent and profound personal growth."

—Rachel Dash, MSW, Faculty Emeritus, West Virginia School of Medicine,
Department of Behavioral Medicine and Psychiatry

"Marseille creates a vivid picture of what it meant to grow up with hearing loss— the complexities, the sadness, the frustrations. Marseille is special and so is her story. She traversed a world that wasn't built for her and in her journey she found her true, authentic self. This is a story you will want to hear for yourself."

—Susanna Storm, AuD, CCC-A, audiologist at Blue Sky Hearing

"A well-written and indispensable book about the author's journey from silence to sound. A must read for able-bodied people to learn about the trials of an invisible disability. This is a heroine's journey—learning to speak, navigating hearing loss, and cultivating other senses for artistic expression—and a testimony to the resilience of the human spirit."

—Theresa Silow, PhD, LPCC, Professor of transpersonal and somatic psychology at the California Institute of Integral Studies

"In her eloquent story of shaping a life as a hearing-disabled person, Claudia Marseille awakens readers to the barriers and biases most of us fail to recognize or fully understand. Through her singular courage, tenacity, and self-discovery she gracefully illuminates the ways difference and determination can transform us all."

—Elizabeth Rosner, author of *Survivor Café:*
The Legacy of Trauma and the Labyrinth of Memory

"Claudia Marseille's memories are reported with vivid color and sight descriptions and muffled sound. This is a tale of medically induced hearing loss, lifelong learning, survival, love, music, and finally art."

—Maureen Fitzgerald, Licensed Professional Clinical Counselor, Certified American Sign Language Interpreter

"Claudia Marseille's beautifully rendered memoir doesn't stop at offering insights into the hearing disabled world. This well-crafted, tender tale begs us to consider the grave challenges faced by the disadvantaged, and how it is that such individuals defy great adversity and champion debilitating handicaps to achieve remarkable personal goals. Marseille's narrative is informative, stirring, and noteworthy."

—Julie Ryan McGue, author of *Twice a Daughter:*
A Search for Identity, Family, and Belonging

"This well-crafted, intimately personal, and honest exploration of the author's truth is a revelatory experience for any reader, whether they are hard of hearing themselves, Deaf, or hearing. In this memoir, Claudia Marseille brings us with her on the lifelong journey of finding her place in the world of silence and sound."

—Ruth Dubin, MEd, CI/CT/SC:L, Nationally Certified American Sign Language Interpreter

"Claudia Marseille's memoir paints an evocative picture of her loneliness and perseverance through hiding her hearing loss during her early life. This is a must-read for new parents, grandparents, pediatricians, and *anyone* who works with children and young people to prevent such isolation."

> —Mary E. McCall, PhD, developmental psychologist, consultant, and
> retired professor of psychology at Saint Mary's College of California

"Claudia Marseille illuminates the experience of living with severe hearing loss in her extraordinary and powerful memoir. With tremendous sensitivity and insight, she eloquently brings the reader into her world of growing up with a serious and invisible disability. My understanding of what it means to live with hearing loss was blown wide open. This needs to be required reading for those in education, healthcare and, simply put, everyone."

> —Miriam Eisenhardt, MPH, RN, Assistant Professor, Samuel Merritt University

"A breathtaking tour de force! Claudia Marseille's heartbreaking memoir is a game-changer, opening new vistas on the world of the hard of hearing. Marseille's sincere narrative seamlessly navigates the gaps between her needs and her reality as she worked hard to create an admirable path forward to the life of her dreams and aspirations. I'm sure I won't be alone in being grateful that Marseille has shared this wonderful story!"

> —Esther Erman, author of *Rebecca of Salerno: A Novel of
> Rogue Crusaders, a Jewish Female Physician, and a Murder*

"Claudia Marseille's memoir recounts her journey growing up with profound hearing loss, mainstreamed in the world of verbal communication. Marseille deftly weaves the realities of the ever-present communication challenges and the deep sense of isolation she so wanted to overcome. We learn just how impactful communication barriers can be. Most importantly, Marseille faced down these challenges and realized her desire to have a fulfilling life and engage as the socially outgoing woman she is."

> —Robin E. Miller, disability rights attorney

"In her compelling story, Claudia paints in fine details the story of her life challenged by a severe hearing loss while also managing to live an adventurous and fulfilling life rich with her many talents in music, art and creativity."

> —Ronnie Wilbur, PhD, Professor, Dept. of Speech,
> Language, and Hearing Sciences at Purdue University

"Claudia's life would be dramatic even if she hadn't been born nearly deaf, but she was, and how she maneuvered with and around her 'disability' makes her account of her life all the more poignantly compelling."

—Noel Holston, author of *Life After Deaf:*
My Misadventures in Hearing Loss and Recovery

"Marseille's memoir was the most authentic depiction I have ever read on this topic. It was so surprising to read about the similarities of our life experiences of hearing loss. Thank you for so beautifully articulating your experience and sharing it with the world."

—Sarah Shapero, MSW, behavioral health counselor

"In this beautifully written memoir, Claudia really hits on the topic of isolation—very common among those with hearing loss. Her vivid descriptions of her colorful journey through complex family interactions, friends, and different professions are truly inspiring as she finally creates a happy and fulfilling life. Her strength and resilience shine throughout."

—Joy Holtzman Antar, MSW, former counselor at the
Alabama Institute for Deaf and Blind/Mobile Regional Center

"A poignant memoir, rich with vivid details about the full impact of severe hearing loss on every aspect of daily life, and ultimately a story of resilience and triumph over adversity."

—Barbara Ridley, author of *When It's Over*

But You Look
So Normal

Lost and Found in a Hearing World

Claudia Marseille

SHE WRITES PRESS

Published 2024
Printed in the United States of America
Print ISBN: 978-1-64742-626-2
E-ISBN: 978-1-64742-627-9
Library of Congress Control Number: 2023917557

For information, address:
She Writes Press
1569 Solano Ave #546
Berkeley, CA 94707

Interior Design by Kiran Spees

She Writes Press is a division of SparkPoint Studio, LLC.

All included images are from the author's personal archive unless otherwise specified.

All company and/or product names may be trade names, logos, trademarks, and/or registered trademarks and are the property of their respective owners.

Names and identifying characteristics have been changed to protect the privacy of certain individuals.

For my husband, Sam Barakat
and
Our daughter, Mira Barakat

For the millions of people
who courageously live
with hearing loss

And for you

Author's Note

I decided to write this memoir when I realized that my friends and even family members had little idea of how severe hearing loss can affect one's life.

My parents chose to mainstream me into the hearing world, and because I didn't meet any other people who were hard of hearing or deaf until my mid-thirties, I had no exposure to ASL or Deaf culture. I was educated in the "oral" method which meant I learned to speak and understand with the vital support of strong hearing aids and lipreading. While I was largely successful with the oral approach, there were significant costs: lack of a sense of community; difficulties in understanding others; and perhaps worst of all, frequent isolation. Because of my significant hearing loss, I felt alone throughout much of my childhood and young adulthood.

My story is about how I navigated two worlds without genuinely feeling I belonged in either one. I didn't fit into Deaf culture, nor did I entirely integrate into a "hearing" and spoken language mainstream culture. As the Deaf world was not part of my experience, in this book I don't describe the richness of ASL and the unique Deaf culture. This memoir is not in any way meant to advocate for mainstreaming or to take a position on the oral approach over the use of ASL and participation in Deaf culture.

In this memoir I refer to myself as being "severely hard of hearing," or as "having a hearing loss," despite that when I was growing up, people used the terms "disability" and "impairment" to refer to my hearing challenges. I have avoided the use of the word "impairment" as the word tends to have a negative connotation in Deaf culture. "Disability," however, is a term that has come into acceptance by many, not only in Deaf culture but among other groups of people with disabilities, so in this story, I occasionally refer to myself as having a disability.

I deeply admire all those who have courageously dealt with the impact of deafness or hearing loss in their lives and have sought to live well despite the many challenges they've had to navigate. I also empathize with parents who have to make difficult choices, including whether or not to mainstream their child. I wrote this book for those who have hearing loss and their families and for the general reader who wants an inside glimpse into one life lived with hearing loss.

Prologue

It was the day of the citywide elementary and middle school track meet, and I was elated that I'd made the cut, one of only two students at our school. At age eleven, I was a good athlete and very fast, and I was thrilled to have the chance to compete against other sixth and seventh graders from across Berkeley. I'd trained hard for this day. For weeks after school my teacher, a soccer coach, drilled my friend Mark and me hard on our school playground, yelling at us to sprint faster, *faster*! Day after day I pushed harder and harder as I raced Mark—the only kid in our school who could run faster than I—and I could feel myself getting better. I also depended on Mark to help me navigate the hearing world. Like my brother Elliot, Mark was very attuned to me. On the playground he faced me directly and clearly repeated what had been said, carefully explaining where we were to line up, how far we'd be running, and who had taken first, second, and third place.

Now standing in the center of the field, I surveyed the bustling scene, and to my surprise I didn't see anyone I knew. Athletes wearing their school colors stretched out on the grass or jogged in place, excited families settled into their seats in the bleachers, coaches with clipboards dashed here and there. My heart thumped in anticipation of the moment when I'd launch from the starting line with the pack of runners, sprint neck and neck alongside other contestants fiercely determined to beat me, and then, finally, stretch into the finish to break the tape. That morning, I fastened my bulky hearing aid with an extra strap to ensure it wouldn't fall off from where it was clipped to my undershirt. I was ready.

I was eager for my mother and father to see how fast I could run, and I looked all around, anxious to spot them in the crowd. Searching the glaring hot metal bleachers, I finally spotted them sitting across the field from each other. Their fraught divorce had left them with no desire to sit together, even to show united support for me. My father looked grim and formal in his dark wool suit, and he wore a handkerchief on his head, each corner tied with a knot, which created a kooky little hat to protect him from the sun. I watched him wipe sweat from his forehead and wondered, *why on Earth would he wear a heavy suit on such a hot day?* Far across the field from him sat my mother, looking cool and elegant despite the sweltering heat, fumbling for something in her purse.

In the distance, I saw a coach yelling instructions into an orange megaphone as sprinters began to line up for races, but I couldn't understand a word he said. I had trained at my familiar elementary school playground, and I was totally unprepared for how the track meet would unfold in this unfamiliar place. I still didn't see anyone I recognized, and I began to panic. Was one of my events just now about to start? Where should I go? *Mark!* I thought. *Mark will tell me what to do, where to go.* Frantically, I whipped my head around looking for him, but he was nowhere to be found. Then, as kids started running, I stood frozen, a little statue in the middle of the field as races whirled around me. Coaches darted about, herding kids and lining up racers. Athletes whizzed past me as they took their places, ran their races, and whooped with joy when they won. But nobody asked if I needed help. No one seemed to notice that for almost an hour I hadn't moved from where I stood rigid on the track.

Finally, it was all over. As everyone streamed off the field, I saw my father in the distance, slinking away through the far exit. My mother was waiting for me by the bleachers, and we walked slowly towards the car. She looked concerned. "Why didn't you run in any of the races?" she asked.

I burst into tears. "I'd no idea where to line up! I couldn't understand the man with the megaphone or what any of the kids were saying."

My mother nodded and murmured sympathetically, but that was the end of the conversation. From the bleachers, both of my parents had sat and watched me just stand there. Why hadn't they run across the field, grabbed me, and guided me to an adult in charge? Why didn't at least one of them recognize that I was in trouble and needed help? And now that the humiliating event was over, there was no exploration of what had happened, why I was so lost, and what might be done to spare me such shame in the future.

As my mother drove us home, I cried quietly in the seat next to her and gazed out the window at the constant activity and clamor that made it so difficult for me to hear or understand people around me. A motorcycle roared in front of us, a bus screeched to a halt to our left, a truck beeped insistently as it backed up on our right. Whenever I was amidst these kinds of city sounds, all I could hear was the tremendous clamor. And most of the time, interior spaces weren't much better; as I sat next to my mother, the rumble of our car made it virtually impossible to understand her unless she turned to face me, which she couldn't do while driving. Tears ran down my cheeks as I realized, once again, how terribly alone I was. Every day I struggled to understand. There was so much I was missing. Meanwhile, almost nobody was listening.

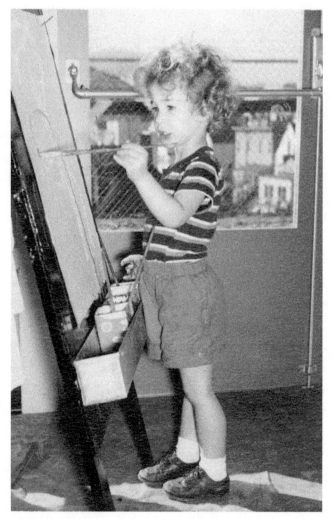

Painting in preschool

Chapter One

My earliest memories are completely silent. Not yet knowing what it was to hear and speak, I'd no idea what I'd been missing, that other people experienced the world differently. As a very little girl, I felt completely at home in my world defined by visual communication and other sensory clues I received through scent, touch, and taste. Silence wasn't a lack or an absence. It simply was—a familiar backdrop to my experience.

Once, when I was about three, I squatted in my grandmother's garden tugging on a weed in the stillness of a late summer afternoon. Light sparkled through the undulating leaves as Omama, wearing a green sweat-stained kerchief tied over her bun, sprayed a glittering mist onto thirsty purple pansies. I ran my fingers through the damp earth, staring with astonished attention at a tiny worm that wiggled its way deeper and deeper into the soil. I didn't hear the warbles of the birds flitting in the bushes, the wind rippling through the trees, or the roar of the airplane soaring overhead. Omama waved to me to come to her, but I didn't hear her calls. All was still. I didn't yet have the words to express it, but that afternoon as I communed with the musty earth, I was aware for the first time of being immersed in a world of pervasive silence.

Later, after I experienced the wonder of sound, I began to better understand silence. Every night after removing my hearing aids, I would reenter the deep and spacious emptiness of a profound quietness. This stillness is a very intimate, palpable experience. Even now I feel it as an inner resonance within my body, and when I resume silence, it's as though I am being enveloped in the warm embrace of a soft, comforting blanket. And each night, I feel the infinite expanse like a starlit night as I lie wrapped in the quiet until morning when I reluctantly emerge to rejoin the world of noise.

But although I've always treasured my nighttime peace, I gradually realized that to be part of the world that rumbled and hummed around me all day, I would have to learn to hear as best as I could. My long journey from silence into sound—with its debilitating lows and intoxicating highs—began in 1950, five months before I was born when my mother was prescribed a seemingly harmless medication to treat her severe nausea.

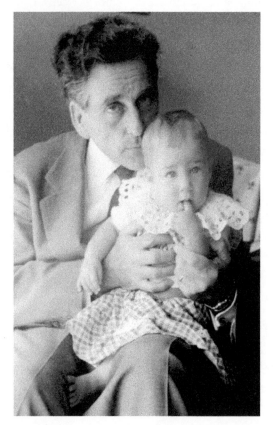

Me with my father

When I was a baby, my parents had no idea I suffered from a severe level of hearing loss. I was their first child, and they didn't notice anything was wrong, despite that by age four, apart from some babbling, I hadn't uttered a word. Most children begin to utter their first words by twelve months, so my parents should have known something was amiss. But they were still adjusting to life in the United States having emigrated from Nazi Germany—my mother shortly after WWII ended and my father just before the war began. Both parents were also distracted by the birth of my brother, Elliot, who was born when I was two. They were busy, but as I'd realize later, they were also in denial.

Eleanor, my nursery schoolteacher, was the first to notice I couldn't hear. She told my parents that whenever she called and gestured for me to come to her, I would obey—if I could see her. But when she called to me from behind, I didn't respond. Eleanor also noticed that I always carefully watched the other children and copied what they did, except during group sing-along. During that circle-time activity, I would rock on a wooden rocking horse, daydreaming while staring out the window at the garden, silently experiencing my own world and oblivious to the singing and activities of the other children. Eleanor suggested to my parents that I should have my hearing tested. My father was outraged and yelled at her, insisting that there was nothing wrong with his daughter. But my mother calmed him down and said it wouldn't hurt for me to be tested.

I was four years old at my first audiology appointment, and I tried to be brave as I walked with my parents into a huge building and then down long halls to a dark, cramped office with a small glassed-in booth. The audiologist was a kind elderly man who squatted down to my level and moved his mouth in funny formations, the way grown-ups seemed to do much of the time. I said nothing and instead lay down and pressed my ear against the linoleum tiled floor. I was feeling the vibrations of the hammering and banging of the remodeling

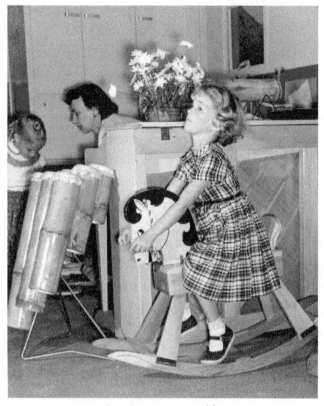

Lost in my own world

taking place in the office below. The audiologist explained to my parents that I was astutely listening for the kinds of sensory clues that people with hearing loss notice but that hearing people ignore. After observing me for only a few minutes, the audiologist suspected I was hard of hearing even before he began the test.

My mother then walked me over to the testing booth and sat me on her lap while I played with my teddy bear. During the test, the audiologist piped in sounds at various pitches and watched to see if I glanced up or tried to identify the source of the sounds. But I just sat on my mother's lap, happily engaged with my bear, not responding to any of the beeps. I also didn't respond when he spoke directly behind me or in front of me. After the test, the audiologist and my parents sat at a table and moved their mouths at each other. All three of them had grim expressions on their faces, so I knew that something serious was going on, but I didn't think it had anything to do with me. I went back to playing with my bear.

The audiologist had my mother's medical records and explained to my parents that I most likely had severe sensorineural hearing loss in both ears, probably due to nerve damage because of medication my mother was given to treat her severe nausea and dehydration during her pregnancy. This medication irreversibly changed the course of my life. He told them that the medication had most likely damaged the developing auditory nerves in my inner ears, a side effect that wasn't known about at the time.[1] He said that I needed to be fitted with a strong hearing aid, immediately, which would help me learn to listen, identify sounds of spoken language, and then speak as soon as possible, as well as prevent further atrophy of the auditory nerves.

Even though I wasn't talking yet or responding when they called to me from behind, my parents didn't notice that something was seriously wrong, so they were stunned to learn how serious my hearing loss was. It was measured and labeled "severe," approaching "profound," particularly in the higher frequencies where many of the distinctive sounds of speech reside.[2]

Later I would learn that the audiologist went on to stress that I couldn't hear my parents speak or sing to me, couldn't hear the music they played on their record player, couldn't hear rattling noises in the kitchen. I certainly couldn't hear rain, birds, dogs or cats, cars, or airplanes. I'd probably be able to hear nearby thunder, he said, but not a siren, which wailed at high frequencies, unless it was very close by. The audiologist warned my parents that even with a hearing aid, I'd most likely have problems discriminating speech, particularly in noisy situations, and he urged that I learn to lipread as soon as possible. My parents asked whether I'd need to learn sign language or go to the School for the Deaf in Berkeley, but he said, "Let's wait and see how she does with a hearing aid."[3]

Two weeks later my father brought home my first hearing aid. My mother and I met him in the street as he got out of the taxi, beaming with excitement. I reached a hand up to my father's, and we walked to our house as I clutched in my other hand my new hearing aid wrapped in a brown paper bag. At home I examined the device with curiosity although I had no idea what it was for. It was gray, about as big as a deck of cards and had a long cord connected to a customized mold that was made to fit snuggly in my ear. My father's enthusiasm was infectious, and I could hardly wait to try it out and show it to my mother and Omama.

I stood patiently in the living room as my father wiggled the mold back and forth in my ear until it fit in place. Then he clipped the hearing aid onto my shirt and turned it on. Right away, I was hit by an explosion of sounds: the painful crack of metal pots in the stainless-steel kitchen sink; the blaring ring of the telephone in the living room; the low, scary rumble of an airplane, its ferocious whine coming from some unidentifiable place in the sky. All this noise frightened me, and at first, I felt completely disoriented as I had no idea where these sounds came from or what they were for. But in the garden a few days later, I saw my father throw his hands up in the air with excitement when he saw me point to birds that were cheeping in the bushes right next to us. At first, I thought the chirps were coming from the bushes themselves, but eventually, to my delight, I registered that the sound coincided with the bird opening its beak. Slowly I began to get used to all the new and unfamiliar sounds coming in through my hearing aid.

Human speech was another story. I was totally confused the first time I heard my family speaking. They had always moved their mouths in funny ways, but I'd never understood why. Now, thanks to my hearing aid, I heard some of what they said, although at first it was all garbled and indecipherable. Over the next few weeks, I learned that the sounds coming out of my parents' mouths meant something important and would help me connect with them.

Within a few weeks I started to utter my first words as my father pointed to different objects and named them: "doll," "teddy bear," "cat," "Mommy," "piano." My first word was "doll." I knew what a doll was by its shape, but now I was learning that the sound "doll" also referred to the doll itself. And if I managed to utter the word "doll," my parents, thrilled, put my doll in my hands. My brain was buzzing with all the new information I was able to take in with the help of the hearing aid; I wasn't only hearing new sounds, I was learning what things were called. But my greatest pleasure came from watching my father's face light up as I started speaking for the first time.

From then on, my father often tested whether I could hear him by crouching down and speaking behind my back ever more softly with each question.

"Claudia, can you hear me? What am I saying? Can you hear me now? Am I saying "cat" or "pat?""

I would turn around to look at his mouth as he repeated the words. I could hear some sounds in the quiet living room, but his voice was too muffled for me to understand what he said unless I could also see his face. I couldn't hear the difference between "cat" or "pat," but by looking at his mouth, I soon learned to distinguish between the shapes of the letter "c" uttered from the back of his throat and the letter "p" formed by his pursed lips. As he observed me carefully watching him, he realized I was relying greatly on lipreading, so from then on, he took care to look directly at me when he spoke. With his help, I could feel myself making great progress, and I was proud every time I heard an excited "Yes!" from him as I came to understand more and more what he was saying. At this point, I was still too young to realize that I was different from others in my family. Mostly I just relished the attention I was getting from my father.

My father thought that since I compensated for my hearing loss by reading lips and facial cues, reading text might be easier than learning to hear and speak. And he was right; I clearly remember the first word I was able to read. Several times a week, we walked up to the blue mailbox a block from our house. He would lift me up to drop his letters into the chute where I would make out the embossed word *Mailbox*. "B-O-X," my father would patiently spell, pointing to each letter.

Then one afternoon when I was almost five, something clicked; sight and sound slotted into place. I realized that B-O-X signified the box itself, and from then on, to my delight and astonishment, I was able to read. At the time I didn't know how unusual it was that I learned to read at such an early age. Understanding what a word meant by seeing it written on the page was much easier than trying to understand speech, so right away, I loved reading time. Snuggling on my father's lap under his thick plaid throw blanket, I would follow along as he read aloud to me from children's books, his forefinger underlining the words. Leaning my head against his chest, I could both hear what he was reading and feel the vibrations of the words from his throat on the top of my head.

Reading exposed me to a world of messages and meaning that helped orient me in my life. From the stories my parents practiced reading with me, like *Grimms' Fairy Tales*, Dr. Seuss books, and the stories of Winnie the Pooh, I learned about the emotions and issues that were common in the lives of children and grownups. My father read with me regularly, explaining what various words meant, and after two years of reading and speaking practice, I could speak in short sentences and read aloud from the Dr. Seuss books. Then I would cuddle under a pile of blankets with my younger brother Elliot and read to him. Reading became an indispensable part of my life.

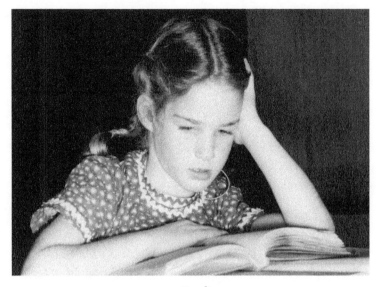

Reading

When I was almost five my family moved from our apartment in San Francisco to a house across the bay in Berkeley, two blocks below the Hillside Elementary School. I loved our apricot-colored stucco house with its castle-like turrets. We each had a room, including Omama, who had lived with us since her arrival from Germany the day before I was born and who was now ensconced in a little suite of her own down a dark hallway. The house had a small lawn in the front with a rose arbor draped over the short path that led to the front steps. Elliot and I splashed about in a cement wading pool situated under a tall, graceful cedar tree. In the backyard was a steep terraced rock garden where I spent many happy hours helping Omama weed and plant flowers.

Inside, three steps led down from the dining room to a large sunken living room with hardwood floors, a room largely devoid of furniture except for a mustard yellow couch, a coffee table, and a dark straight-backed wooden chair that enthralled me, its legs carved in the shape of gargoyles. In a corner of the room sat a baby grand piano that friends of my parents had passed on to us.

Throughout that house, I discovered new places and ways to learn how to hear. I sat for hours on the piano bench, my legs swinging back and forth, dreamily sounding out notes and savoring the different pitches of the tinkling tones. During lazy afternoons, I lay on my sunbeam-splashed bedroom floor, watching luminous fairy dust motes gently swirl about me as I pressed my ear against the speaker of my little record player. Again and again, I listened carefully to the only words I could discern: "Oh my darling, Clementine." I couldn't get enough of the music, and I wondered who Clementine was.

When I was five and Elliot was three, I realized that my brother wasn't like me, that he could hear and understand in ways I couldn't. We were building a block tower in his room when I heard a faraway, unclear yelling sound coming from our mother. I didn't understand the words, so I ignored the sound, but my brother turned to me and said clearly, "Dinner time!" I realized then that she'd yelled a message and that Elliot had translated it for me. And like my father, Elliot also learned early on that he needed to look at me when he spoke. Soon I depended on him to explain what transpired during family conversations at home, in the car, and while playing outside with children in the neighborhood. He became the first of many people I relied on throughout my life to interpret the world around me, and this reliance knit me closely to him.

In time I began to understand that as important as it was to be able to hear, sometimes silence had its advantages. One evening, as I stood outside my parents' bedroom, I could hear the doors slamming and my father shouting in German. My mother, not wanting me to witness one of their fights, hustled me away, tears staining her cheeks. I turned my hearing aid off, letting the silence surround and comfort me, dissolving the tension in the house. In time it became a habit to turn my hearing aid off during their frequent fights.

But turning off my hearing aid was not just for tuning out con-flicts. Silence also helped me focus enough during one incident to save my little brother from injury, maybe even death. One Sunday when I was five and Elliot was three, my mother drove the three of us across the Richmond Bridge to Marin County for a hike on Mt. Tamalpais. My father rarely accompanied us on outings, and this day was no exception. It was early spring, and the world glimmered a vibrant green. We clambered up a hill, and then Elliot and I sprinted ahead across a flat expanse of meadow which—although none of us knew it at the time—ended abruptly at the edge of a steep cliff overlooking the ocean. We ran headlong toward the horizon but then suddenly slipped, tumbled, and landed on a narrow ledge six feet below the meadow's edge. Looking down, I saw that we stood on the crumbling side of the cliff just above a perilous decline. The ledge was the only thing between us and the steep drop to the sharp rocks far below.

I could tell by my mother's frightened expression as she peered over at us that Elliot and I were in danger. She lay flat on the ground, inched her way to the edge of the incline, and stretched out her arms to pull us back up, but Elliot was just beyond her reach. She yelled panicked instructions to me, which I couldn't understand. My first thought was that I had to protect my precious hearing aid before I could help Elliot. I took it off, tiptoed along the ledge, and carefully passed it up to my mother who wordlessly took it from me. Then in the silence, I was able to focus on rescuing my little brother. Kneeling next to him, I grabbed his ankles and guided his feet into footholds, then slowly pushed him up the cliff as he climbed step by step into our mother's outstretched arms. Finally, she reached down and pulled me up. Crying with relief, she hugged us both to her, and I felt a surge of confidence course through my body. By staying calm and grounded I'd been able to extricate myself and Elliot from danger. The quiet had allowed me to do that.

I was always very protective of my hearing aids. Gradually I was learning how important they were, that they connected me to my family and that without them, I'd be alone in my own isolated world. So even from my earliest days, I never lost or damaged one of my hearing aids. But ironically, while my hearing aid connected me to others, sometimes I needed to tune out the barrage of sound they delivered to better focus. By instinctively taking my hearing aid off as I clung to that ledge, I was able to shut out my mother's frantic voice and just concentrate, trusting in myself. It's a practice I continue to this day, periodically turning my hearing aids off when I need to focus. Sometimes eliminating sound makes it easier for me to attend to what's important.

A few days after the incident on Mt. Tamalpais, my mother, smiling mysteriously, led me by the hand into my room. Sitting on my dresser was a resplendent green parakeet in a shiny wire cage. Ever since the first time I'd heard the birds chirping in the bushes, I'd dreamed of owning a pet bird. My mother beamed as I threw myself into her arms for a hug, wondering if this new pet was a reward for helping rescue Elliot. I named my new companion "Peter" and spent many hours with him, pressing my face close to his cage as I tried to teach him to talk—hoping he could read my lips as I read to him. I taught him to sit on my shoulder where he nuzzled my neck, chewed on my hearing aid cord, and pecked at seeds I held out in my hand.

I was allowed to release him from his cage only when it was being cleaned or when an adult was present to make sure he didn't escape my room. But sometimes when no one was watching, I'd let him out so he could sit on my head and squawk in my ear, keeping me company while I played with my dolls. I adored Peter, my first pet.

One afternoon I hosted a tea party for my dolls and stuffed animals, and I wanted Peter to be part of the festivities. I released him from his cage, and he happily flapped around the room. Then he perched on a curtain rod, gazing with heavy lids down at me and my dolls, but soon I forgot all about him. By evening, I remembered I'd let him out of his cage and was terrified to discover he was nowhere to be found. Panicked, I ran to my mother. I was relieved she wasn't angry at me for letting him out, and she suggested we leave his cage door open and put a slice of apple in his food dish, hoping to entice him back in. But Peter didn't show up.

The next morning, as I was making my bed, I pulled the bed from the wall, and Peter fell with a dull "thunk" onto the wooden floor. Horrified, I realized he must have been stuck between the wall and my bed, desperately cheeping all night long for help. Clutching his limp body to my chest, I wailed at the thought that my lack of hearing might have caused his death. And even though my mother didn't reprimand me, I felt the horrible weight of guilt for having let him out to roam freely and for not having been able to save him. Peter's traumatic death led to a frightening realization: My lack of hearing could be dangerous.

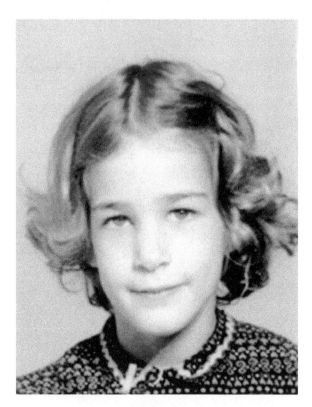

Kindergarten

Chapter Two

"In school you'll learn to read books and think for yourself," my father told me. And although I was excited to begin kindergarten and "learn to think" at Hillside Elementary School, I was more concerned about learning to speak like everyone else. I was already able to read, but I was just beginning to talk in short sentences, so I began weekly speech therapy and lipreading practice with Mrs. Christiane, the school speech therapist. This therapy would continue for the next seven years.

Mrs. Christiane was a sweet grandmotherly woman with gray curls, and I relished the dedicated attention she gave me. Throughout elementary school I was pulled out of class for an hour every Friday to work with her in a small office stuffed with plastic toys and a medical model of the mouth, tongue, and throat that sat on a low table. When Mrs. Christiane nodded and smiled to indicate that I'd made a sound correctly, I tried to memorize the feel of the sound in my body, how I had used my throat and shaped my mouth and tongue.

The cognate pairs were tricky; it was hard to tell through lipreading the difference between the voiceless "p" and the voiced "b," and the nasal "m." Same with the "t" and "d" and the "f" and "v." And then there were the sibilants, which in the language of phonics refers to sounds made with a hissing effect: the "z's," "s's," "sh's," "sch's," and "ch's." Being in the high frequency range where my hearing loss was most severe, these sounds were simply too soft for me to hear. Over and over, I had to practice placing my tongue and forming my mouth in the right way to execute these phonetic challenges.

Mrs. Christiane would ask me to look into a mirror to see how we shaped our mouths when we made a certain sound. As we worked, I was mesmerized by her tongue with its deep groove in the center which waggled as she enunciated the letters. She would place my hand on her throat or my palm in front of her mouth so I could feel the vibrations of the different airflows produced by the sounds. We spent a long time focusing on the subtle differences between the "ch" in "church" and the "sh" in "should" and the "sch" in "school" until one day I felt a forward release of air in my mouth when I articulated "sh" as opposed to a vibration when I made the sound of "sch." After years of concentrated effort focusing on Mrs. Christiane's mouth to articulate different sounds correctly and consistently, I was finally getting the hang of it. I was excited to make these distinctions which I could feel with my hand placed on my throat, and I was proud when she regularly rewarded my accomplishments with a gold star sticker and a hug.

Later, in fifth grade, I played weekly games of gin rummy with my new speech therapist, Mr. Scott. To sharpen my lipreading skills, he would silently ask me questions about school, my friends, and what I was going to do for the weekend, and soon I excelled at reading his lips. Years later, my mother told me that Mr. Scott used me as a case study in presentations about how lipreading can be an effective addition to hearing aids.

In elementary school, I was self-conscious about the way my bulky gray hearing aid bulged heavily beneath my shirt or dress. In the mornings, my mother helped me clip it to my undershirt or place it in a little pouch secured with straps over my shoulders, across my chest, and around my back so it wouldn't be dislodged while I was playing. The bulge was very obvious and made me think I looked like a robot. My classmates teased me for having some kind of square breast in the middle of my chest, and sometimes a child yanked out the plastic cord that snaked conspicuously around my neck to the customized mold in my ear. The yanking hurt, and I'd have to persuade my classmate to hand the mold back to me. Then, I'd carefully work it back into place in my ear.

In kindergarten during one recess, I saw some girls tittering in a circle, pointing at me as I hung upside down on the monkey bars. I mustered my courage, swung down to the ground, and walked up to them.

"Are you a Martian?" Marsha teased. I was afraid of Marsha, a ringleader who was bigger and older than the rest of us and who sometimes beat up little kids. She planted herself squarely in front of me and was fingering my hearing aid cord. The other girls crowded closely behind her, and my heart began thundering in my chest. I had seen a Martian in a comic book, and I certainly didn't want to be seen as weird, but I took a deep breath and answered her. "No," I replied, "do you want to try my hearing aid?"

Marsha held out her hands. "Be careful," I said as I nervously fished the device from inside my dress and placed it in her outstretched hand, hoping she wouldn't drop it. I was excited to show her my hearing aid, and I held my hand steady as I raised the mold up to her ear. One by one, the girls jostled each other, eager to try it out. They smiled at me as they carefully held the mold up to their ears. But because the mold didn't fit their ears, the hearing aid screeched its loud feedback whistle, which to my relief they treated like an interesting toy.

Most of the girls didn't actually experience hearing sounds amplified, but that playground demonstration seemed to satisfy their curiosity and diffuse the mystery and strangeness about me and the unfamiliar contraption I wore everywhere. Before long, we scattered to play a game of tag. By the next day, word of my show-and-tell session got out, and during recess the boys lined up to try on my hearing aid. They were more inquisitive, spending more time with it during their turn and asking whether they could have one too. I was hugely relieved that everyone was so interested, and I was pleased I'd had the courage to show it to them. Their acceptance made me feel just a little less different.

After most of the kids had experienced my hearing aid, the issue of my being different was more or less forgotten, and I wasn't teased again on the playground. But my two days of show and tell didn't mark the end of my school social troubles. Often, I felt separate because I just didn't know what people were talking about during group conversations. When I couldn't understand a game's complicated instructions and rules, I stood alone, lost on the playground. The other kids were too busy playing to notice my awkward confusion, and I felt invisible, surrounded by the swirl of kids and games all around me. I desperately wanted to be included, and it was only during my mid and later elementary school years when I had a best friend who explained the rules that I could wholeheartedly participate in the recess games.

I loved my kindergarten's art and sewing class, which relied on seeing rather than hearing. For one project, we drew and cut the shape of a hen out of stiff cotton fabric and patiently hand-stitched the two pieces together, leaving a little opening of about two inches. Then we turned the form inside out, stuffed it with cotton balls, and sewed the little opening shut. With crayons, we colored the body of our hens yellow and gave them red beaks. I gave mine blue eyes and red cheeks. Proud of my hen friend, I napped every afternoon hugging her to my chest.

One afternoon, I took my hen home to show to my mother, and it was on that day that I first understood that my parents' marriage was having difficulties. She murmured admiringly and said, "Let's show it to Daddy." We went upstairs into his study where my father sat hunched over his desk, and she held the hen out to show him.

"Look what Claudia made in kindergarten," she said in a cheerful voice. But he just continued to write, his back turned to us. He

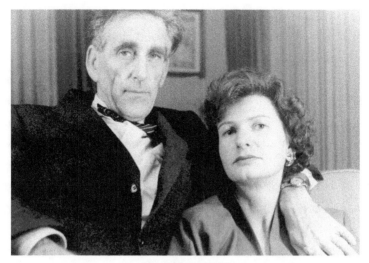

My parents, 1955

didn't look up or say anything. Crushed, I thought I'd done something wrong—maybe we shouldn't have entered his study without knocking. But my mother led me out of the room, looked down at me, and said, "He's angry at me, so he won't talk to either of us. It has nothing to do with you."

"Why's he angry at you?" I asked.

"It's too hard to explain."

I was confused and wanted to ask her more questions, but she turned her face away from me, placed her hands on my shoulders, and steered me downstairs into the kitchen for a snack of cookies.

Over the next few days, my father continued to refuse to speak to my mother. One evening as we sat together around the dining room table for dinner, instead of asking my mother to pass the butter, which was right next to her, he said to me, "Ask your mother to pass the butter." At first, I thought this was a fun game, but after a while, as I watched their grim faces, I didn't like it anymore. To break the heavy silence hanging over the family dinner, Elliot and I shrieked and kicked each other under the table, but Omama tried to shush us as the tension around the table only thickened with our antics. We finished the meal in silence with Elliot and me nervously giggling as we bussed our dishes.

I didn't like our father's bizarre and erratic behavior, but as children often do, I simply accepted the way things were and became used to his moods. Several weeks passed, and my father still wasn't talking to my mother. It was Halloween, and I wanted to go out dressed as a queen. My mother had sewn me a glittery silver dress with a sequined silver and gold cape, and on the day of Halloween, she helped me make a crown of gold foil and fastened it to the top of my blonde curls. I had also lost a front tooth that afternoon and was excited to show my father my beautiful costume and the gap in my teeth. Again, my mother and I went upstairs to his study, this time knocking on his door. I entered the room shyly, eager for my father's approval of my royal attire.

"Look at Claudia's costume. Doesn't she look beautiful?" my mother said.

But again, he refused to look up or say anything to either of us. I was crushed and confused. He also didn't join us when our mother took Elliot and me trick-or-treating with the other kids in the neighborhood. I noticed other fathers out trick-or-treating with their kids and I missed his presence.

By Thanksgiving, my father was finally talking to my mother again, but by Christmas he was back to living in stony silence. The atmosphere his isolating grimness created in our home was oppressive; my mother and Omama were quiet as they went about the house, their faces drawn. Omama tried to distract me by asking me to help bake Christmas cookies. I adored her and loved to help her bake. As we did every Christmas, we made her favorite cookies from her childhood in Prague: lebkuchen, zimsterne, pfeffernuesse, and a large yeast stollen. She helped me roll out butter dough on the wooden breakfast nook table and press out star shapes with a cookie cutter for the sugar cookies. Beaming at me with her bright blue eyes, she allowed me to scatter multicolored sprinkles onto the cookies and lick the rich, creamy dough off the wooden stirring spoon. I came to associate the ritual of baking alongside Omama with a certain magic of the Old World she embodied. She helped create a homey and loving atmosphere in an otherwise tense household, and I cherished her for it.

That Christmas, my father decorated our tree without saying a word to my mother. On Christmas Eve, he lit the candles on the tree, which was resplendent as usual, adorned with gold tinsel, red apples, and tangerines. In addition, he hung the carved wooden ornaments that my mother had brought with her in her suitcase when she emigrated from Germany. For my first Christmas, my father had carved for me a small wooden mouse, which he painted blue with yellow ears and a red snout, and every year he would tuck the mouse deep in the tree on one of the pine branches for me to find. On that Christmas Eve when my father wasn't speaking to my mother, I raced to the tree to hunt for my mouse as my brother ran over to his pile of presents. I looked over to where my mother sat quietly on the sofa watching, and I hoped she would also have some presents to open, but there was nothing by her chair. As I opened my presents, my heart grieved for her as she watched the rest of us tear open our surprises. But there was nothing I could do, and I tried to put my parents' difficulties out of my mind as I played with my toys.

The tension between my parents only added to the insecurities I already struggled with. I was afraid that my father no longer loved my mother and worried that he might leave us. They argued in German, so I couldn't understand what they were fighting about, but I could hear and feel the tone, and the arguments often left my mother in tears and my father in stony silence. My father's unkindness caused me to feel a split between my love for him and a dawning realization that he was simply mean, mean to my mother and to me by way of his silent treatment. I felt torn; I was protective towards my mother, but I didn't want to acknowledge this unkind part of my father. I also took his meanness personally. He didn't seem to realize or care that by punishing her he was also punishing me. At not quite age six, I couldn't reconcile the idea of my sometimes attentive, fun father also being this man who could behave so coldly for weeks at a time.

Omama saved that difficult Christmas Eve for me and helped me forget my mother's pain. She pointed to a present wrapped in gold tissue paper and topped with a pine frond, which she'd tucked among my other presents. As she watched me open it, her face glowed with excitement. It was a Kaethe Kruse doll with long blonde braids, and it wore a pale blue dress imprinted with white stars.

"She came to you specially, all the way from Germany," Omama said. Germany, I imagined, was a fairy-tale land of magic and mystery.

"Her name's Dora," I announced to the room. Clutching the doll to me, I climbed onto Omama's lap and threw my arms around her neck. She held me tight, and I tried to sit for a while, but she was short and rotund, so it was impossible for me to sit on her lap for long without sliding onto the floor. She kissed the top of my head, murmuring "*Schatzie*," which I knew meant "treasure," and then released me to play with Dora.

The next day was Christmas, and Omama suggested we invite all my stuffed animals and other dolls to a resplendent tea party to meet Dora. She crouched with me at my little table while we wrote elaborate invitations on paper doilies sprinkled with gold glitter. Over the next few afternoons, we combed my dolls' hair and dressed my dolls and stuffed animals in their most elegant clothes. Omama hand-sewed a few magenta-colored capes for those animals who had no special clothes to wear, and we set out my dolls' china teacups in a big circle on the floor of my room on a tablecloth made of colorful scarves. We then decked it with pine branches, crystals from Omama's collection, and crimson rose hips from our winter garden. The animals and dolls arrived in their stagecoaches, which I fashioned out

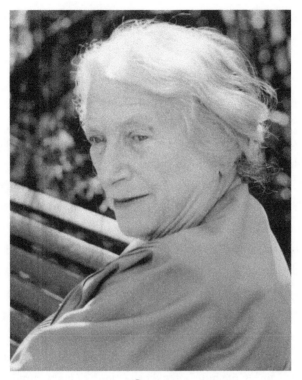

Omama

of wooden cars, and Omama, opening the door to each coach, formally introduced them to Dora. Omama, who had been a well-known actress in Germany, impersonated different voices for each animal in her broken English, and I was enthralled. Dora was gracious, serving everyone tea and desserts, and the party ended with lively dancing. Our little event was a great success, and my heart swelled with love for Omama and for the chance to forget my parents' troubles.

Shortly after that Christmas, I turned six, and to my great relief my father started talking and paying attention to me again. Every few months he would descend back into one of his dark moods, but for much of the time I had my fun-loving father back. I was very excited to start piano lessons, which both my parents encouraged, and I was delighted when my father would practice with me as I learned to read music. When I would repeatedly stumble on the same wrong note, he would jokingly call the mistakes "ooblecks" after Dr. Seuss's *Bartholomew and the Oobleck,* the story he read to me over and over about a boy who tries to rescue his kingdom from a sticky green substance that spreads into everything. He told me I should try pressing my fingers lightly and quickly on the keys so I wouldn't get stuck in the oobleck.

One afternoon my father positioned himself at the piano, his hands hovering above the keys. I waited at the top of the three steps that led down to our sunken living room and flamboyantly stretched my arms out until I heard him strike some dramatic opening chords. He nodded up at me that it was time to make my entrance. Swirling my glittery silver and gold Halloween queen's cape about me, I descended the stairs, flapping my arms and then pranced, whirled, and pirouetted across the room.

"Can you hear the notes? Can you tell what they are?" he asked, playing a chord while hunched over the piano to make sure I couldn't see his fingers on the keys.

"I can hear you. You're playing. F, A, C, F in both your left and right hands," I answered, skipping across the room.

"What about this?" He was excited, I could tell. He played another combination.

"In your left hand you're playing E-flat, B-flat, G, and E-flat. In your right hand it's just E-flat and G," I rattled off.

Ever since learning music, I had associated the notes with specific colors, and I could see the different colors as my father played the various chords. Middle C was a rosy pink in the middle of the rainbow of my imagination. The F below Middle C was a dark blue, and the F above Middle C was a lighter blue. For me, notes simply corresponded with colors, and it was easy to tell what the notes were. I just thought this skill was common.

"And this?" My father hunkered down farther over the keys, again making sure I couldn't see his fingers. This time the task was more difficult; I could hear he was hitting some dissonant notes, and those were harder for me to discriminate. "B-flat, C, E-flat, and F in your left hand. And I think E-flat and F in your right hand," I answered, hesitantly.

"You're absolutely right!" he exclaimed. He played a few more chords, and each time I'd announce their notes correctly, he'd become more enthusiastic.

"Let's try the doorbell." He walked outside and pressed the button to our front door. "Can you tell me what these tones are?"

"That's easy. It's a G and then it goes down to an E flat."

He strode back across the living room to the piano and played those notes to check for himself the interval of the doorbell and said, "That's right! Amazing! And what about the ring of the telephone?"

He walked over to his office phone line and dialed, then watched me expectantly as I listened to the telephone ringing.

That was easy too. I was able to call out the correct notes, and I beamed up at him with pride.

"You know, you're very hard of hearing, but you have perfect pitch. That's *amazing!* It's very rare," he explained. "Most musicians have good *relative* pitch—that means they need a first note to guide them, and then they can tell what the other notes are. But you don't even need that first note. It's remarkable!" He dashed off to tell my mother and Omama about his discovery, but I didn't understand what all the fuss was about as the pitches of various sounds were obvious to me. I couldn't imagine not knowing what the notes were because I clearly saw all of them arrayed on a rainbow with each note's color lighting up as that note was sounded.

Later I'd learn that this ability to see what one hears is a form of synesthesia, experiencing one of your senses through another. Over time, I no longer saw the rainbow; I just knew which note I was hearing. It was, I thought, just as anyone can tell that an orange is the color orange or that the sky is blue. To me, it was as simple and familiar as knowing which way is home. In time, I came to understand how unusual absolute pitch is, but back then, I simply loved all the attention I was getting.

When I was seven, I became friends with Linda, who lived two blocks away. I loved playing with her in her basement recreation room, which was devoted entirely to all the toys she and her brothers owned: dolls, stuffed animals, a large electric train set, and a rocking horse. I was especially drawn to her big doll, which had flaxen hair tied back in a pert, bouncy ponytail. She generously let me take her home for a whole week to play with. Linda and I became close, and she was the first of many friends who explained the rules of the games we played with other children. This became very useful as Elliot and I would meet up to play with the other neighborhood kids—Kip, Alex, Martin, and Gordon—nearby at the cul-de-sac where Gordon lived. Linda and her brother, Butchie, and their elegantly coifed gray poodle Cinnaboo often ran down to join us, and I was always relieved whenever she arrived, as I relied on her for help with the games.

Because of the shape of the cul-de-sac, we kids called ourselves the U-gang, and out in the street we played kickball, hide-and-seek, red light/green light, and tag until the sky turned purple. With all the yelling back and forth, I often had no idea what we were playing, especially if Linda wasn't there to tell me. But then, usually, Elliot would notice when I seemed confused and would explain what was going on. Although he was two years younger, he was protective of me, and I relied on him to explain the dynamics of the gang. In turn, I looked out for him when older boys in the neighborhood surrounded him, ready for a fight. I was turning into a scrappy tomboy, and I would yank off any boy that pounced on Elliot.

My parents didn't own a television, so Elliot and I joined the other kids of the U-gang early on Saturday mornings at Martin's house to watch Looney Tunes. But because the cartoons were animated and the animals' mouths were distorted, I couldn't read their lips. Sprawled in a heap on the floor, the other kids squealed at the animals' various antics, but I couldn't follow the story lines.

At these television gatherings, it further dawned on me that I was different. I knew I had a hearing aid and that other people didn't, but I was beginning to understand that the hearing aid was to correct something that was missing. I now associated my hearing loss with my difficulty understanding television shows and connecting with kids in a group, in the school cafeteria, and during games. I realized that these were all situations where it was difficult to discriminate speech from the background noise, and this realization led to a painful sense of deficiency and separation that became more and more familiar as I grew older. Often the other kids didn't notice that I didn't understand them, and this just added to my sense of isolation. Sometimes I envied Elliot and other children who were free to connect with an ease that they took completely for granted. Unlike in kindergarten when I was willing to have everyone try my hearing aid on, now I tried to pretend I *wasn't* different. This unconstructive practice of trying to hide my hearing deficit to fit in continued through my adolescence, and it only served to make me feel more left out.

That Christmas my father asked me to help wrap a present for my mother. I was excited to see what he'd bought for her and hoped it would be something special, like a diamond ring. Not that she had ever mentioned wanting diamonds, but my friend Ellen's mother had a large diamond ring, and I was dazzled by its glittery flashiness. From witnessing my parents' fights and my mother's tears, I knew that my mother was unhappy, and I desperately wanted her to be happy. I thought a big shiny diamond would cheer her up, and I was crushed when my father proudly showed me his present for her: a pewter pin of a lion with an outstretched paw and a flowing mane. No diamond ring. No necklace encrusted with jewels. Nothing sparkly or spectacular in any way. I was sad for her, but I didn't say anything, hoping that by some miracle the gift would be meaningful to them and make them a happy couple again.

"Let's wrap it up extra special," my father said. My parents had recently bought a new refrigerator, which had come delivered in a gigantic cardboard box. My father dragged the box up from the basement and deposited it in the middle of the living room.

"We'll wrap the present in bigger and bigger boxes and end up with the refrigerator box, so it'll be a real surprise for her," he said.

I was torn. I was excited at the idea of using the refrigerator box. But I was also nervous that the pin wasn't special enough for such an enormous container. Even though I was only seven, I was concerned how this was going to turn out. My father hung a big sheet over the entrance to the living room and instructed my mother not to come in while we were working. First, we wrapped the pin in its little jewelry box with gold paper and a filigree gold ribbon. Then we went in search of another slightly larger container. I gave him the box that I used to hold my prized collection of different-colored lucky rabbit foot charms. We placed the gold box with the pin into that box and then wrapped it in silver paper with a purple ribbon. Next, we found an empty shoebox and continued the process. This continued all afternoon as we wrapped the present in still larger and larger boxes; in the end, we used nine boxes until we finally wrapped the refrigerator box with newspaper. As we wrapped all those boxes, my father became increasingly animated, but as he became more flamboyant, I felt my heart constricting more and more. I feared that after going through the effort to open all those boxes, my mother wasn't going to love the gift inside. I wanted to help bring my parents together, not be part of something that would disappoint her.

On Christmas Eve, my parents lit the candles on our large fir tree, and we listened to German Christmas carols, "Heilige Nacht" and "O Tannenbaum" on the record player. Then my father turned to my mother and said, "It's time for you to open your present!"

She flushed with excitement and curiosity as he whipped off the sheet covering the huge box wrapped in newspaper with a large red bow. She smiled with elation as she opened the first of the packages, but after unwrapping a few boxes she grew frustrated. At one point, she even let out an exasperated, "Ach, Valter." I perched on the arm of the couch, hanging over my mother's shoulder to be able to hear her when she finally opened the small box with the pin inside it. "Oh, how pretty," she said. But I could tell from her flat voice and the way she avoided my father's face that she was disappointed. Once again, I was heartbroken that my father couldn't make my mother happy. I worried about how her unhappiness would affect my parents' marriage and our family life.

Chapter Three

By the time I was in third grade I was aware that my father wasn't like other fathers. On weekdays he worked at home in his study but rarely at his profession as a psychoanalyst. Although he had an office in a refurbished room in our basement where he saw patients, my mother told me he had very few of them. One afternoon after I saw one of his patients leave his office, I went down to look for my father. He was standing at his metal file cabinet putting away some papers, and he waved for me to come in.

"What do you do in here?" I asked, flinging myself down on the chaise that was normally reserved for his patients. I rested my head back against the small Persian carpet that lay draped over the top of the chaise and stared at the whimsical Miro print on the opposite wall.

"I help my patients understand their relationships with their parents," he explained in his typically formal way of speaking. "They learn about this from how they behave with me. They act out with me what they really want to do with their parents. For example, a man might be really angry at his father and want to kill him. But this is an unacceptable thought, so instead he behaves badly towards other people, even though it's really his father he hates. This is called *projection*. Patients need to work out their Oedipal issues of love and hatred with their parents."

"What does *Oedipal* mean?" I asked.

"If the child is a boy, he falls in love with his mother and wants to marry her. He's envious of the attention his mother gives his father, so he wants to kill his father. And if the child is a girl, it's the other way around."

I found this all very disturbing, the idea of marrying one's mother and killing one's father. I swore to myself I would never project anything on to anyone, ever. The adult world seemed so complicated, but I liked that he talked to me about grown-up things.

One afternoon a few days later as I was practicing the piano, my father flung open the front door and staggered into the house under the load of several cardboard boxes and plunked them down on the bottom of the staircase that led to his study. He waved for me to come over and look. The boxes were filled with hundreds of booklets with the title written in big letters, *The Walter W. Marseille Mail Order Rorschach Test*. He knelt down and fished out a booklet to show me.

"What are these?" I asked. I was impressed to see his name boldly printed on what looked like a very official publication. I flipped through one and saw it was full of pictures of symmetrical abstract images, some in black and white and some in color.

"These pictures are formed from inkblots made on a folded sheet of paper," my father explained. "The Rorschach test offers a way of seeing whether someone is emotionally disturbed. If they are paranoid or crazy in their thinking, this test will reveal it. Remember when I explained to you the very important idea of projection? People will project their mental health issues onto what they see in these images."

"Did you paint these pictures?" I asked, pointing to one I particularly liked, a red, black, and white image of what looked like dancing fairies touching hands.

"No, they were made by a very intelligent man, the Swiss psychologist Hermann Rorschach. When I trained in Berlin to be a psychoanalyst in the early 30s, I was also trained to administer this test to patients to identify what their problems were. Now your daddy wants to do these tests on people throughout America, so I'm going to send these pamphlets out to clinics and hospitals around the country."

I listened, enthralled, sitting cross-legged on the bottom step while he paced back and forth on the landing.

"Patients will write down what kind of animals or objects they see in the pictures and then send the booklets back to me. I'll analyze their answers and write back to them and explain what their issues are."

"Are you the only person in the whole wide world doing Rorschach tests?" I asked.

He sat next to me on the step, wrapped his arm around me, and pulled me close. I rubbed my cheek against the rough tweed of his charcoal gray suit. "No, I wish I were," he said. "It's become a very popular test. But I'm the only one doing mail-order tests. It cost me a lot of money to have all these pamphlets color-printed, but I'll make lots and lots of money from this. You just wait and see. Your daddy is a very clever man, and soon people will know about me. I will become famous. And your Mami will see this too."

My mother was always worried about our family's finances, and her worries flowed down to me. "How are you going to make money from this?" I asked him.

"People will send me a check for my diagnosis of their problems."

I ran to my mother to show her one of the booklets, but her lips were clamped tight as she nodded slowly. My mother's negative reaction dampened my hope that this idea of my father's was going to work out. Not for the first time, it was hard to reconcile my father's extreme exuberance with my mother's pessimism; my loyalty towards my parents continued to be painfully split.

But I relished the next few afternoons as he administered the test on me, writing in meticulous detail in a notebook what I saw in each of the inkblots. He conducted the test three times to see if my answers were consistent. I loved being taken so seriously, and I was proud as he nodded at my answers: "a crab," "two women sitting back-to-back," "a scary moth," and "two playful dwarves pressing their hands against each other." *I must be doing this right,* I thought, as he beamed his approval at me.

Over the next several evenings, I helped my father at the kitchen table by pressing stamps onto the booklets as he carefully hand-addressed them with his fountain pen. But after a few weeks, although I checked every afternoon, I never saw a single test returned through the letterbox at the bottom of our front door. Eventually I stopped hearing about the Rorschach tests. Like his wrapping my mother's Christmas present in the refrigerator box, another of his lofty ideas didn't go as he'd hoped. Even as a young child, I could see that many of my father's ideas were larger than life and didn't turn out well. Again, I was torn between wanting to be supportive of him and feeling shame at his failed ventures. I felt embarrassed for him although he himself didn't seem to be embarrassed; he just continued to busy himself with more projects.

I wished my father worked like other fathers. Most of the time, while my mother was busy attending classes at UC Berkeley, working towards a master's degree in social work, and Elliot and I were at school, my father practiced his opera singing, worked on the techniques of archery, or played tennis, bocce ball, or chess. On the side, he was writing a book about Sigmund Freud and Karl Marx, but this project had been going on for many years with no end in sight. Mainly he spent time on the complex Japanese board game called Go, in which players use stones to try to surround each other's territory on a checked board. Most days, he spent many hours playing Go by himself. He'd taught himself enough Japanese to follow the games played by masters, which were printed in specialized Japanese Go magazines for students to follow, and he regularly traveled across the Bay Bridge to Japantown in San Francisco to compete in tournaments against highly-ranked Japanese Go players. One day he proudly told me that he'd just been seeded as the number one non-Asian Go player in the United States, but I wasn't impressed; I just wanted a father with a regular job.

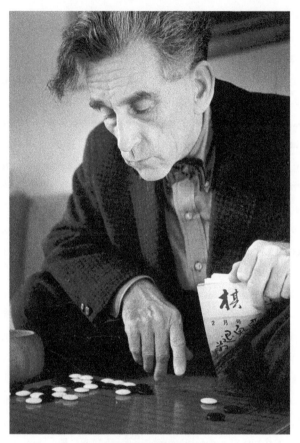

My father playing Go

One afternoon I peeked into the study where he sat stooped over the wooden coffee table holding a white Go tile between his second and third fingers and gripping a Japanese Go magazine in his left hand. I checked his expression to see if he was in one of his grim moods. Sure enough, his look of concentration in mid-play meant I could under no circumstances disturb him, so I waited in the hallway by a reproduction of Bruegel's "Fall of Icarus" that hung at the top of the staircase. I loved studying that painting while waiting to be allowed to enter my father's study. I never grew tired of spotting Icarus's legs flailing above the water; I was fascinated by the boy who splashed headlong into the sea after ignoring his father's warnings not to fly too close to the sun.

After twenty minutes, I carefully peered again into my father's study. Disappointed, I saw that he was still studying his Go magazine. Finally, he placed his tile with a decisive click onto an intersection on the board. At last, he stretched his arms out to me, and I dove into his lap and pressed my cheek against his chest. For those few moments, I relished the security of being enveloped in his arms and forgot about my worries about his not working.

But many times as I walked home from school, I'd hear him bellowing opera exercises out the window of his study—"EEOooh EEOooh EEOooh EEOooh Yoooyh!" I was ashamed that my father was not at work like other fathers, and I was embarrassed at his strained and cracked voice. He didn't seem to care that the whole neighborhood could probably hear him. When I walked home with other kids, I didn't want them to connect this strange man to me, so I'd walk down the street past our house, and then, as the other kids peeled off into their homes, I'd weave my way back up my block.

One hot afternoon in late spring, as I was walking home with kids from the neighborhood, we approached my house, and I slowed down at the sight of my father standing on the sidewalk across the street from our house. Wearing a white T-shirt and tennis shorts and with sweat streaming down his face, he was shooting arrows onto a target on our lawn. As the other kids edged away from him, I stopped and watched as he posed like some aging archer out of a Robin Hood story. He took careful aim at the big round target that was stuffed with straw and positioned on a tripod in the middle of our lawn. He stretched back the bowstring and launched a long metal-tipped arrow. Even from where I stood, I could tell that those sharp arrows were made to penetrate flesh, not straw. *Thwack!*

Humiliated, I could hear the other kids murmuring things about my father, but I couldn't understand what they were saying. After standing a moment to study his most recent shot, he reached his arm back, plucked out another arrow, positioned it against the string of his bow, drew back his arm, and then waited, motionless and ready as clusters of children cowered on the sidewalk behind him. Then another *thwack!*

I looked up and saw neighbors glaring down from houses along the street, but my father kept on, as if he were the only person outside that day. Soon, I heard the screech of sirens, and I watched, my cheeks hot with shame, as two police cars skidded up to our house. My father talked quietly with the police, then slowly crossed the street back to our house. I bowed my head low and hurried down the street pretending not to see him. Later at home he never mentioned the incident, so I never knew if he, too, had pretended not to see me. I knew this was not the way fathers were supposed to spend their workday. It was hard to reconcile my split heart—my love for him and feeling completely mortified by his behavior.

At first, I didn't want a party for my eighth birthday, but my mother insisted I have one. I'd rarely been to a party that included anyone outside of the family and was afraid, because of my hearing limitations, I wouldn't be able to handle the socializing involved with having a group of friends over. It was very hard for me to follow a conversation with several people talking at once, especially when the speaker didn't look directly at me. I told my mother I was worried about being the party's hostess, but she said, "Oh, you'll do fine," so the decision was made. *But she doesn't know what it's like with a group of kids,* I thought. *I might be left out at my own party.* That was my worst nightmare. But I kept it to myself.

She sat me down at the dining room table, gave me eight invitations, and told me to decide who should be on the guest list. While I

was at it, she suggested, I could practice my handwriting by address-
ing the envelopes. Because I had trouble socializing in groups, I didn't
have many close friends, but I was able to think of eight girls from
school and the neighborhood to invite. I spent the afternoon at the
dining room table sprinkling glitter inside the envelopes, and then
carefully block printing their names and addresses. I was very pleased
with how artistic and colorful my invitations looked, and little by little
my fears about the party began to ease. My father told me he'd mail
the invitations the next day, and I watched as he placed them in the
inside pocket of his heavy tweed overcoat.

The next day, my mother took me to Birdie's toy store in downtown Berkeley where, to my delight, I was allowed to pick out party
favors: multicolored party hats, sparkling pinwheels, bags of marbles,
rabbits' feet, and blowouts with fringes. Back at home, I placed these
items in rainbow-colored party bags that I labeled with each girl's
name. When I was finished, I went into the kitchen where my mother
was cooking dinner and asked, "Can I have a chocolate cake from
the Virginia Bakery with lots of frosting and eight pink roses?" My
mother smiled and said, "Yes." My heart swelled with love for her.

Despite my fears about socializing in a group of chatty girls, I
was excited about the party. I was hoping to make some new friends
and be included in the existing group of neighborhood girls. After
two days, I asked my mother if she'd heard back yet from any of the
girls' mothers. She said it was too early, that the invitations probably
hadn't even arrived in their mailboxes yet. But after eight more days,
my mother still hadn't heard back from anyone, and I could tell she
was worried. Eventually she told me, "Something's wrong. I haven't
gotten any RSVPs." She couldn't figure out what could've happened.
But I knew: Nobody wanted to come to my party.

My mother called my best friend Ellen's mother to see if she
had received the invitation. She hadn't. My mother then called the
other mothers and found out that none of the girls had received

my invitation. Finally, after a search, she found the invitations still inside my father's overcoat; he'd completely forgotten to mail them. I was devastated, and I saw my mother sharply reproaching him in his study as he sat hunched over his desk. He didn't look up or say a word to either of us. Once again, my father hadn't come through. He wasn't trustworthy. I was crushed that he couldn't be bothered to mail the invitations to a party that meant so much to me, and I felt betrayed.

My mother called all the mothers back, explained what had happened, and invited their daughters. It was short notice, and I was sure that everyone would say "no" because now they all had an easy excuse to avoid spending time with me.

"Everyone wants to come," my mother assured me, "but some have already made other plans. But still, it'll be a nice party." Now I was even more anxious. I wasn't sure that anyone really wanted to come to the party, having convinced myself their mothers were forcing them into it.

The next day, I put on my white lacy party dress, and my mother tied plaid maroon and pink satin ribbons on the ends of my braids. Sharon, Pat, and Alex arrived right on time, similarly dressed in fancy white dresses and handed me presents wrapped in colorful paper. Ellen was the only remaining "yes" who hadn't yet arrived, and as the four of us stood awkwardly in the landing waiting for her, I tried to strike up a conversation with the others but had no idea what to say. They chattered amongst themselves, but I couldn't follow their conversation. One of my biggest fears was coming true: I was being left out of my own party.

Finally, the doorbell rang and I rushed to open the door for Ellen. She stood at the entrance elegantly dressed in a flouncy copper-colored taffeta dress with an ivory lace collar, a dress that made her seem much more sophisticated than the rest of us in our lookalike white dresses. She entered the house and held out a large present wrapped in gold paper. I was so happy and relieved to see her, but then I noticed that her eyes were swollen and red from crying.

"What's the matter?" I asked.

"I got in trouble with my father. He got mad at me, pulled down my underpants, and gave me a spanking. He wanted to punish me by not letting me come to your party, but my mother said I had to come."

She was sobbing and I was shocked. Her father was strict, and I'd always been a little afraid of him, especially after I'd once seen him roar down the hall and grab Ellen's twin brother for a spanking. But now I felt her humiliation. My father, for all his difficult moods and erratic behavior, would never do something like that.

I took Ellen by the hand and led her into the dining room, which my mother had decorated with pink and light-blue crepe garlands draped along the ceiling. I sat her down next to me. My mother, apparently oblivious to Ellen's plight, came out from the kitchen beaming as she carried my chocolate cake with its eight pink roses. Everyone joined in singing "Happy Birthday," and I blew out the candles in one breath. I opened my presents while the girls sat in a circle on the floor around me and looked eagerly on. I was thrilled with Ellen's present, a set of paper dolls with elaborate costumes from around the world, and I smiled broadly at her. But Ellen just looked down at her lap. I didn't know what to say to my best friend, who was usually very bubbly and often helped me in social situations but was now locked in her own private anguish. Also, I couldn't understand the other girls who talked and giggled amongst themselves; I was lost and miserable. My mother, not noticing my distress and awkwardness, smiled as she bussed the dishes and busied herself picking up wrapping paper.

We played a few rounds of pin the tail on the donkey and then whacked at a piñata—both were games that were easy for me as they didn't involve talking. Finally, after a couple of hours when it was time for everyone to go home, I was relieved. I loved my beautiful cake with eight roses, but the party created too many stressful moments that I didn't know how to navigate. At last, I could return to the quiet cocoon of my home life where I didn't have to struggle to make it through a mysterious social terrain. Finally, I could go to my room and play with my paper dolls.

Three years later when I was eleven, I had another birthday party, a slumber party that also didn't go well. I couldn't hear or lipread the girls whispering in the dark once the lights were out, so once again, I felt excluded from my own party. Thoroughly miserable again, I decided that group parties weren't for me and that from then on, I would socialize with only one friend at a time. I wanted desperately to fit in with my peers and their group dynamics. But in the years that followed, I'd learn just how difficult it would be to make that wish come true.

Chapter Four

I loved being eight. By then, I was fully immersed in the thrill of reading and had proudly transitioned out of picture books. I was independently reading all of L. Frank Baum's *Wizard of Oz* series, many of the *Nancy Drew* mysteries, *The Secret Garden*, *Little Lord Fauntleroy*, and *Juan and Juanita*. Elliot and I relished the times our father read to us. One of the books we most loved experiencing with him was *Rascal* by Sterling North, the achingly sad memoir of a boy's relationship with his family and his pet raccoon, and we loved that our father affectionately nicknamed us his "rascals" after North's raccoon.

We never tired of hearing him read *Winnie the Pooh*, and I especially loved *The Little Prince*, a story about a downed pilot's relationship with a lonely prince he meets in the Sahara Desert. The prince describes his feeling of exile as he journeys through the universe and has interactions with the one lone adult residing on each planet he visits. I could relate to the loneliness and isolation of the prince.

"Rascals," our father said to us one evening as we were listening to him read *The Little Prince*, "notice how Saint-Exupéry makes fun of the adults in the book." He wanted to make sure we understood these references to adult pretensions and vices, their power plays and need for admiration. I loved that Saint-Exupéry, along with our father, recognized a certain wisdom in children, our ability to see through hypocrisy and make fun of grown-ups; even more, I liked that my father thought we were clever enough to see through the narrow-mindedness of adults.

Our father also introduced us to Charles Schulz's *Peanuts*. He brought home paperback books of *Peanuts* cartoons, and after school we cuddled up next to him on the living room sofa as he read to us of the various adventures of Charlie Brown, his dog Snoopy, Lucy, Schroeder, Violet, Patty, and Pig-Pen. We couldn't get enough of these cartoons with their vignettes of sweet relationships between friends, between boy and dog, between siblings. My brother and I caught the humor, and our father made us feel grown-up by discussing the stories with us like peers.

"These cartoons are so much better than any of the others out there," he said. "Schulz really understands what it's like to be a child. He shows us children's true feelings, including their hatred and jealousy—not just their nice feelings." I could relate deeply to the messages in Schulz's cartoons. My experiences of being excluded were validated by his stories, and I loved him for it.

Within my family, Elliot had the best grasp of the impact of my hearing disability. Often left to our own devices while our mother attended the university and our father labored over his various speculative projects, my brother and I were nominally supervised by Omama, although by now we were too rambunctious to pay her much heed. Elliot and I were fast companions and played together with our toys, balls, and board games, and we created our own games like "fort."

One afternoon we pulled the blankets off our beds and draped them over my little table and chairs. We were hiding from Native Americans, and Elliot had his cap gun at the ready in case of an attack. I always hated when he played with it because the blast of the cap firing was excruciating for me. Unlike modern hearing aids, early hearing aids had no ceiling on the level of amplification; it was the same across different frequency levels, so loud noises were always very painful.

"Ow, that hurts! Warn me when you're gonna fire the gun!" I said.

A few minutes later, Elliot said, "An enemy is sneaking up on me, and I'm gonna fire my gun now." I was then able to quickly turn my hearing aid off before the blast went off on his gun. I was grateful for his understanding and his warnings. And out in the neighborhood as we played with other kids, I continued to rely on him to explain what was going on. We were very close.

As we crouched in our fort, Omama flung the blanket door open and handed us hot lemonade mixed with honey and a plate of cookies.

"You need nourishment if you're going into battle," she said.

"Oh, thank you, angel of mercy," we cried out, arms outstretched as she left the room with an amused smile. But shortly after, we got into a fight and rolled on the floor, punching each other and yelling. Omama charged in and sent Elliot back into his room, but within five minutes we became bored and quietly tiptoed to the landing between our rooms and stretched our arms out towards each other. We recited our make-up chant of nonsense words that we used to patch up our fights. Soon the rancor between us was forgotten and we got back to the serious business of playing.

Despite my hearing disability, I loved school. I was good at sports and reveled in playing kickball, red light/green light, and capture the flag. Because I was a good athlete, I was always one of the first picked for teams, and the thrill of being chosen went a long way towards making up for the times I was left out of social groups. But most of all, I loved the structured work of the classroom, particularly reading, spelling bees, vocabulary quizzes, and handwriting.

My father had told me that I needed to work on my vocabulary, that I didn't use as many big words as other kids my age. He explained that my limited speaking vocabulary was due to my not hearing many of the words used in normal conversation, even though I understood many "grown-up" words from my reading. To please him, I wanted to catch up. Miss Magnuson, our bubbly teacher who had short blonde curls and wore cat eyeglasses, black with gold sequins, handed out mimeographed sheets of words and their definitions every Friday, which I diligently memorized for the quizzes on Monday mornings. I was highly motivated to do well, to be seen by everyone as a good student, and to my great pleasure, I always aced the Monday morning quizzes.

But best of all, one afternoon my block printing was deemed neat enough that I was allowed to graduate from using a pencil to a ballpoint pen. When Miss Magnuson handed me the Palmer cursive handwriting book, I could barely contain my excitement. I felt very grown up as I dove into learning the artistry of cursive script. Practicing my handwriting was meditative and peaceful, and it made me feel like an artist.

However, during social interactions on the school playground when I didn't have a best friend by my side, I often stood adrift and invisible, not able to figure out how to be part of the other girls' conversations and games. I watched as girls strolled in pairs along the perimeter of the playground, their arms hooked around each other's waists, whispering to each other. They would pass by me without even a glance, and I realized with a leaden sorrow that I was missing out on something important.

As the years went on, my mother became stricter with me. I knew she wanted me to be a good German daughter. I was a bit of a tomboy, which she didn't mind when I was outside playing, but she didn't like it at all when I argued or contradicted her. By now, I hated when she sometimes insisted I wear dirndls, the Alpine Bavarian dresses that her best friend Maria had sent from Munich. I particularly hated the floral apron that went with a dirndl; no one else in my school wore outfits that looked like costumes, so I'd hide my apron behind a bush on the way to school. After school, I'd fish it out of the bushes, brush it off, and put it back on just before reaching home. I also didn't like the satin floral ribbons my mother tied in big bows onto the ends of my braids, so I took those off too. I was having enough trouble fitting in without complicating my situation with dirndls and satin bows.

I also couldn't fit in during my dance classes. On Monday afternoons, I walked from school to the legendary Greek-inspired "Temple of the Wings" for the expressive dance lessons my mother had signed me up for. The temple was a fantastical building nestled high in the Berkeley Hills and had been designed by the well-known local architect, Bernard Maybeck. It was complete with arches and Corinthian columns and an outdoor stage for dance performances. The lessons were taught by Sulgywnn Quitzow in the free-form modern dance style of the famous dancer, Isadora Duncan. My mother enthusiastically explained that Mrs. Quitzow was well-known in Berkeley for having brought Duncan's interpretive style of dance to the United States.

One Saturday afternoon, my mother took me to a performance given by the older students. Fascinated, I watched them twirling about on the stage in their sheer rainbow-colored flowing robes and togas. They flew like magical fairies and sprites, and I sat immobile, entranced. I wanted to join them in their dance under the swaying eucalyptus trees and could hardly wait until I, too, was good enough to perform on stage.

But after a couple of months, my dance lessons lost their appeal. Mrs. Quitzow would call out various animals that we were supposed to imitate through our movements. With her back turned to me as I whirled and leaped about on the circular dance floor, I couldn't understand her as she spoke. And the sound of the piano made the situation even worse by drowning out her voice. That, plus the other students' whooping and hollering, made it impossible for me to hear her instructions. So usually I'd wait, watch what the other kids were doing, and then copy them, always a few steps behind.

During one class, as I pranced across the wooden floor lost in my world—we were being fairies, I thought—I noticed that everyone else was creeping and writhing on the floor. Embarrassed as the other children looked up at me, I dropped to the floor and began writhing as well. After a few more classes in which I was similarly lost, I told my mother I didn't want to take any more lessons, that I thought the dances were silly. I didn't want to tell her the real reason I wanted to quit because I wanted to protect her from the full impact my hearing loss had on me; I didn't want to witness her disappointment in my limitations. Out of a loyalty to her, I wanted to be as normal as possible.

When I told her I wanted to give up the dance classes, I was relieved that she just nodded and didn't ask any questions. But I was also sad that I'd never get to wear one of those multicolored silk dresses and dance amongst the columns in the outdoor theater.

I intentionally withheld from my mother how lost I was in the classroom and in groups, and this holding back began a pattern between us: Rarely did I tell her about my struggles, and because she often didn't anticipate the situations that would be challenging for me to navigate, she didn't or couldn't intervene. I believed there was nothing she could have done for me anyway. Equally important, admitting my disability to her would make it more real for me; I was protecting myself from acknowledging the full impact of my hearing loss.

There was plenty my mother couldn't protect me from, including some of the dangers of the outside world. One late afternoon when I was still eight years old, Linda and I were the only children left on the school playground. As the sky unfurled into a lavender sunset, we were playing tetherball, which I loved because I was good at it, able to jump high and punch hard so the ball snapped quickly round and round the pole, high out of Linda's reach. From the corner of my eye, I caught sight of two tall men in their twenties tossing a basketball into a hoop nearby. They were watching us as well, but mostly I ignored them until they came over and started to talk to us. I couldn't understand what they were saying, which made me feel insecure until I heard one of them ask if we wanted to play Doctor. A feeling of dread washed over me; this I didn't want to do. I didn't know exactly what playing Doctor meant, but I suspected it would involve taking off our clothes like when we removed the clothes from our dolls when we played Doctor with them.

The men grabbed our wrists and marched us across the playground to an area behind the school that was thickly covered with overgrown bushes where we kids played hide-and-seek. I was frightened. I looked over at Linda, but she was staring straight ahead. She seemed frozen, not wanting to look at me or at the men. Playing Doctor with strange men didn't feel right, but I was paralyzed with fear and didn't struggle against the tight grip on my wrist. Instinctively orienting myself, I took a mental note of the bungalow down the hill off to the right where I had gone to kindergarten.

The men led us past some trees and then sat us down next to some bushes in a little clearing. It was too dark to see well, and I couldn't get a good look at them. Frozen, I stared down at my shoes; they were my favorite pair, gray Hush Puppies that were good for running races. Linda was also looking down. Then, finally, I looked up and saw the taller one unzip his pants and put his hand down his front while the other one was talking rapid fire, saying things I couldn't understand. I knew we needed to escape, so I grabbed Linda's hand and we sprinted through the scrub toward the kindergarten bungalow. There was a wooden fire escape ladder fastened to the side of the bungalow, and we scrambled up onto the flat roof and pressed ourselves onto our stomachs. Linda silently pointed to the bushes swaying side to side as the men hacked their way through them looking for us. Then we watched as they made their way to a parked car nearby and sat inside. Lights flickered as they lit cigarettes.

Although I was scared, I also felt triumphant, high and hidden up on the roof. We lay motionless for what seemed like an hour as the sky turned a deep indigo blue, and we watched as the stars gradually spread across the heavens. Eventually, the men drove off, but still we lay there. A police car pulled up and parked nearby, and two policemen searched below us with flashlights, occasionally calling out although I couldn't understand them. It didn't occur to us that they were looking for us. We were afraid we'd get in trouble for being so late, but we waited for what seemed an eternity until the police car eventually drove off. Finally, Linda and I clambered down from the roof and separated to run to our homes. As I approached my house, I was surprised to see a police car parked on the street, lights flashing. Inside the living room my father was talking in a hushed voice to two large policemen and my mother was in tears. When I walked through the door, she jumped up and grabbed me, enveloping me in a tight hug.

"Where *were* you?" she demanded.

"Two men took me and Linda to the bushes to play Doctor with us," I said. "But we ran away and hid on the bungalow roof."

Seeing my father's stony face, my mother in tears, and the police—so official looking—in the house lessened my sense of invincibility. Everyone was taking this very seriously, and I realized that something really bad could have happened to me. Once I told them I wasn't hurt, they didn't ask anything more about what had happened in the bushes. They wanted a description of the two men, but I couldn't give them one.

What kind of doctoring the two men had wanted to do with us was a mystery to me, but I knew it had to be bad when they took us to a hidden spot and the one man unzipped his pants. As I had sat there in the dark with the two scary grown men, I'd been close to tears, but thinking about it later, I felt proud of my instincts that took over and got us to the safety of that rooftop. We had saved ourselves by outwitting adults.

Several times over the next two weeks, the elderly school secretary ushered me out of class and sat me down at a table in the principal's office where a young blond policeman showed me a thick album of mug shots. But I never recognized any of the men.

A few weeks later I asked my father if the police had ever found the men. "No, they never did," he said.

My parents didn't talk further with me about the incident, but they did institute a new rule: I had to be home from the playground by five o'clock when the playground emptied out. They bought me a watch with a Mickey Mouse face so I could tell the time. I was pleased with my new watch, but it reminded me of the danger that girls seemed subjected to more often than boys. There was a mystery to men that I didn't understand or want to think about, and I wondered if boys were subject to the same perils.

My sense of power and security in the world was rattled, exacerbated by my hearing disability. My inability to hear what the men had been saying made me realize how vulnerable I was to dangers at the hands of others. And though I didn't know it at the time, my self-protective instinct had guided me to become an even more careful observer of body language and facial expressions. I realized that people said a lot without using words, and I began to sense that my intuition and vigilance would help keep me safe.

Chapter Five

"Do you know what evil looks like?" my father asked. I shook my head. I wasn't sure I even knew what the word *evil* meant. It was Christmas Day, and I was almost nine years old. We were headed up the two blocks from our house on LeRoy Avenue to my elementary school, and I pushed the heavy new bike I'd gotten for Christmas. My father was going to teach me to ride it on the playground.

Although I badly wanted a bicycle for Christmas, I was disappointed because this bike was painted a matte blue rather than the glossy red I'd hoped for. Worse still, it had fat wheels, which I knew would make it difficult to ride in the hills of Berkeley; it would never go very fast. But as my father was so enthusiastic about the bike and because I didn't want to appear ungrateful, I pretended to be excited about it. I did love the metal basket in front, and I was pleased that the bike's bell, which rang shrilly with a press of my thumb on the lever, was loud enough for me to hear.

It was a brilliant, razor crisp blue morning and there was no one else out on the street. I was thrilled to have my father all to myself. As we approached the school surrounded by tall, graceful cedar trees I looked up and said, "Tell me about evil." He reached into the pocket of his brown tweed herringbone coat, took out his worn leather wallet, and pulled out a red stamp with foreign writing. There was a man's face on it in a three-quarter profile, severe, with a short mustache and circles under his eyes.

"This man was very, very bad. His name was Adolf Hitler, and he was pure evil. He killed millions of Jews in Europe during World War

II and destroyed Germany and nearly destroyed the world. Look at this picture very closely, Claudia, for you'll never see anyone more wicked than this. He built concentration camps where he used poisoned gas on the Jews, people with disabilities, and his political enemies."

"What are concentration camps?" I asked. He told me that Jews were forced from their homes, crammed into boxcars that carried them to prisons where they were starved, frozen, and then shot next to graves they'd been forced to dig themselves. Some had been gassed to death with poison that was piped into large shower rooms.

"*Why*?" I asked, distressed. The adult world was much scarier and more complicated than I ever could've imagined.

"Hitler and the Nazis hated the Jews. Hitler thought they were bad people, subhuman even. And he wanted to make more room beyond Germany for the German people to take over."

"Mommy and Omama are Jewish. Did he think they were sub-human? Did he try to kill them?" I asked. I also wondered if I would have been considered disabled enough to be gassed too, but I didn't want to ask.

"Yes, if they could've, the Nazis would have killed Mami and your Omama too. They had to hide from the Nazis in Munich and in the countryside during the war. And Mami had to pretend she wasn't Jewish."

Nazis. Even the word sounded scary. On the verge of tears, I imagined men, women, and children packed naked and screaming into a shower stall, suffocating from the poison gas. I had so many more questions, but then my father said, "Well, that's enough of that. Let's teach you to ride your bike."

We were now at the top entrance of the school playground. He showed me how to mount my bike, told me to pedal fast, and then gave me a starting shove. I took off, pedaling fast as he told me, but it wasn't hard enough, and soon I careened out of control like a spin-ning coin wobbling from side to side. Then suddenly in front of me I spotted a stooped elderly woman with a cane shuffling slowly across the playground. To my dismay, I realized I didn't know how to turn or stop; my father had forgotten to teach me how to brake. Frantically, I rang the shiny new bell with my thumb, but it was too late. I crashed into the old woman, knocking her onto her side, her glasses clattering across the asphalt. My father ran over to help her up. She was confused and shaken, but fortunately she and her glasses were all right. I whimpered as I had scraped both knees, but mainly I was frightened by our conversation about concentration camps and because I'd just knocked over an old lady with my bike.

"Why didn't you brake?" my father yelled, and I shrank into myself. He'd never yelled at me before, and I didn't have the nerve to tell him that he hadn't taught me how to stop. That was the end of the bike-riding lesson. We slowly walked the old lady to her home nearby, her hand clutching my father's arm.

When we got home, I didn't tell my mother about the Hitler conversation. She soothed me as she gently put Band-Aids on my scraped knees, then I made my way to Omama's little suite. On the way I peeked into her linen closet to see if I could find the stash of M&M's she kept hidden in a tin box below her folded white nightgowns. Sometimes she would sneak M&M's or lemon drops to me and Elliot, instructing us not to tell our mother. But this time there were no candies in the box.

As I left the hallway, I found Omama sitting at her desk writing a letter in German, her fountain pen scratching across a sheet of translucent paper. When I entered the room, she looked up and beamed. "My Schatzie," she said, folding me into her arms and kissing the top of my head. My hearing aid screeched from the feedback caused by her pressing my head against her bosom. Although I treasured the affection, I never liked it when she or my mother's friends hugged me that way because of the piercing whistle. I pulled away and showed her the Band-Aids on my knees, but I was too mortified to tell her about knocking over the old lady. She kissed my knees and said, "Now they'll be all better." I plunked myself down on her bed and wrapped myself up in her gray faux fur throw blanket.

"Did you have to hide from the Nazis?" I asked.

She winced but answered me directly. "Yes, your mami and I had to hide in Munich during the war. After the war, your mami left Germany and moved to San Francisco where she met your daddy." My father was German but not Jewish, she explained. He had emigrated to the United States just before World War II because his anti-Nazi activities—his involvement in a resistance group in Berlin—made it too dangerous for him to remain in Germany.

"Then in 1950 when your mami was pregnant with you, she wrote to me and suggested I come and join them in San Francisco. You know, I was so sad because so many people in my family died in the concentration camps during the war. Your mami thought perhaps I could start a new life in the United States." I decided not to ask her about the concentration camps; I had a more important question.

"Were you excited to see Mommy again?"

"Oh yes," she said. "I was very excited to see your mami again. I hadn't seen her for four years since she left Germany, and I wanted to be there for your birth too! And you know, I took a propeller plane, my first time in an airplane. It made many stops for fuel in the United States before landing in San Francisco. And then do you know what happened? Your daddy picked me up at the airport and brought me to the apartment in San Francisco. Your mami took one look at me, and the next morning you were born!" I smiled at the love radiating from my grandmother's blue eyes. I threw my arms around her in a tight squeeze and then ran to show off my Band-Aids to Elliot.

But I couldn't tell Elliot about Hitler, nor could I shake off the heaviness of hearing about the concentration camps and Omama and my mother having to hide during the war. My grandmother had always talked about the beauty of the German landscape, and it seemed to be where fairy tales, magical presents, and cookies came from. But now I was hearing about an ugly side of Germany, and I was confused. The three people I loved most came from a country that had committed unthinkable atrocities. How could that be? I was having a hard time holding the contradictory feelings I now had for Germany: love and fear. I wished I hadn't heard about evil.

That spring I was subjected to a betrayal by my father that further tore at my loyalty to him. Our relationship was already strained because he'd forgotten to mail the invitations for my eighth birthday party. This new rift began during a Sunday afternoon picnic. The five of us had found a lovely spot in Tilden Park in a meadow surrounded by a green collage of tall eucalyptus and oak trees, toyon and manzanita bushes, and tall grasses that rippled in the wind. The warm air carried the aromatic scent of the bay trees down the hill. Omama, plump in a light blue dress with white polka dots, and my mother, graceful in a green sleeveless blouse and white pedal pushers, spread out the blue and white plaid picnic blanket and laid out ham slices, potato salad, pickles, and fruitcake. My father had brought along his bocce balls to practice playing, although we soon discovered there wasn't a flat enough spot anywhere in the meadow.

Once the food was laid out, he jumped up and said to Elliot and me, "Give me twenty minutes so I can turn into a coyote and hide in the woods. See if you two rascals can find me."

"How'll we know where you're hiding?" Elliot asked.

"You'll have to look for my clues and figure them out. There's a very big, very grand prize if you can find me."

After eating lunch and waiting twenty minutes, Elliot and I whacked our way through the thick underbrush and struggled to make sense of his cryptic messages penned in his distinctive handwriting on little slips of white paper pinned onto various bushes.

"Walk twenty feet south, then turn east and walk another ten feet. Then look between your legs and up at the sky," said one clue.

We had no idea where south or east was. It didn't occur to us to look up at the sun to orient ourselves. Periodically Elliot heard our father in the distance, howling a coyote-like *Ow-Oo-who-oooh* in his operatic voice and yanked my arm to go off in the direction of the sound. I, of course, couldn't hear his coyote howls, so I just followed Elliot. After what seemed like hours, Elliot and I still hadn't found him, so we returned to the picnic area where my mother and Omama sat on the blanket eating in grim silence. When my father finally emerged from the bushes covered in dirt, his thick black hair wild with leaves, we packed up the food and drove home. No one spoke. Elliot and I, disappointed, didn't dare ask what the grand prize might have been. My mother was withdrawn; Omama and my father were expressionless. I imagined that Omama and my mother were resentful for having had to wait all that time when we were supposed to be having a family picnic.

The next morning, I woke up covered from head to toe with a blistering rash, particularly on my face and eyelids. By the evening, my eyes were glued shut with a goopy white pus from poison oak. My mother gently bathed me in cool water and covered me in calamine lotion, which cracked off as I brushed against the sheets in bed. Later, examining my unrecognizable puffed face in the mirror, I thought, *I look like a monster.* I missed school for ten days.

A few days later, as my mother tenderly soaked my eyes open with lukewarm water, she relayed how, when I was six months old, my father had laid me naked on my baby blanket in a patch of poison oak. My parents had been attending a luncheon in Mill Valley given by one of my father's psychoanalyst colleagues. At one point, my father excused himself from the cocktails in the living room, lifted me from the bassinet in the guestroom, and carried me outside to the undergrowth in the back garden. He decided to conduct an experiment—perhaps, if I were exposed early to poison oak, he thought, I would develop an immunity. I didn't get poison oak during that first exposure as a baby, but clearly I didn't develop an immunity because by the time I was eight years old I'd already had several severe outbreaks just from brushes against bushes during walks in Tilden Park.

Ten days after the picnic, my father was supposed to look after me while my mother was attending classes at UC Berkeley. Instead, he sent me back to school in the middle of the day and drove across the Bay Bridge to Japantown in San Francisco to compete in a national Go tournament. I still felt quite sick, looked horrible, and I didn't want to go back to school. As I dragged myself into my third-grade class-room, I cried, the salt from my tears stinging the sores on my face. My teacher, aghast, asked me a question while my classmates whispered amongst themselves. But I couldn't hear what my teacher asked and so without saying a word I slowly shuffled to my seat. Ashamed of my face and my tears, I put my head flat down on my desk; I felt betrayed that my father would send me to school looking like this.

Later that evening when my father returned from San Francisco I stood outside my parents' bedroom and listened to them shouting in German. Miserable, I realized that playing Go was more important to my father than my feelings and that I couldn't trust him to put my best interests first. As much as I loved him, I couldn't rely on him to take care of me the way my mother did.

Soon we were all subjected to another one of my father's grandiose schemes. Over dinner one evening he announced, "The rose arbor will have to be ripped out to make room for a bomb shelter on the front lawn." I had no idea what he was talking about, but I was scared at the thought of bombs. The next day at school, Ellen, who often explained what was going on with the adults around us, told me her parents said the Russians might start World War III. "We're all going to burn up and die. My parents said we're gonna turn into toast," she said as we crouched together under our desks, clutching our hands together. It was the Cold War, 1959, and we were used to an occasional duck-and-cover drill, but this morning the teachers seemed particularly upset.

Why would the Russians want to bomb us? I wondered.

That evening my father explained that the Soviets had just shot down an American U-2 reconnaissance jet that had been on a spy mission flying over Soviet territory. President Eisenhower claimed that the aircraft was just a weather plane, not knowing that the Russians had already captured the pilot and had gotten a confession from him. Khrushchev presented the pilot as proof that the American president was lying.

"This is a dangerous situation," my father explained. "Now neither side can trust the other. The Cold War's getting hotter."

"But I thought you liked the Russians," I said, confused. "Remember when you were all excited about the Russian Sputnik and you let me stay up late and we tried to find it orbiting in the sky?"

"That was different. That was a major scientific achievement." he said. "The Sputnik was a huge blow to America's morale, and now we're working hard to catch up with the Russians. Russia and America are in a race to become the most powerful country in the world. Both countries have very powerful weapons, so the situation is very scary. The Russians may try to bomb us." His face was drawn and I was scared.

The following evening I sat with him at the kitchen table and helped him write a list of things we'd need for our bomb shelter. We'd have to buy cases of canned food, enough to stack to the ceiling. "And can openers too," I added. And we'd need mattresses and sleeping bags for five people, plus flashlights, candles, and matches. My mother always walked out of the room during these discussions about the bomb shelter.

"And what about hearing aid batteries? What if I run out while we're in the shelter, and I won't be able to hear anybody?" I asked.

"Good thinking," my father said. "We'll have to buy some extra batteries." He sketched the floor plan, indicating where we'd all sleep and the trap door that would open to the stairs leading down below.

We'd have to rent a bulldozer to dig a big hole, and he calculated the amount of concrete that would be needed. I was concerned with lots of details. "Will Omama be able to make it down the steps?" I asked. *How're we going to pay for all this? And what about the radiation after the blast?* I wondered.

One evening a couple weeks later, my parents were dressed to go out for a rare dinner together in San Francisco, my father handsome in a dark suit and maroon bow tie, my mother smiling, elegant in a navy blue dress. As I hugged her I could feel her girdle and the clips that held up her stockings. My parents looked beautiful together, and I was thrilled to see them outfitted so exquisitely for a night out. I so wanted my mother to be happy. Maybe my father would change and act more normal now.

The next day I saw the sketch for the bomb shelter in the wastebasket in my father's study. To my relief, the bomb shelter, a source of discord between my parents, wasn't mentioned again. But a few months later, out of the blue, my life changed dramatically.

It happened on a Saturday when Elliot and I had gone over to play for the day with our friends Toni and Leonard. Like my mother, their parents were also German Jews, and we had met their family at the Sierra Club camp in the Sierra Nevada mountains the previous summer. I liked Toni. A year older than me, she was a lot of fun and I looked up to her. At the camp we waded in streams, built dams, balanced on logs, and wove daisy chain wreaths that we placed on each other's heads. She taught me how to hyperventilate by pulling a paper bag over my head, and we spent hours in her tent trying to pass out while her parents and my mother were hiking in the mountains. As usual, my father hadn't come with us on that vacation.

That evening, after our mother picked us up from playing with Toni and Leonard at their house, and as she pulled out of their driveway, she blurted out, "Daddy and I are no longer happy together, so I've left him. You kids and I are moving to a new house. I'm going to divorce your father."

From my position in the back seat, I couldn't understand what she was saying, her eyes focused on the road in front of her, but I sensed it was momentous news. Elliot turned to me and explained what she'd said.

"What about Omama?" I wanted to know right away. "Where'll she live?" A cold numbness dragged through my body.

"Omama's coming with us. She's waiting for us at the new house."

"Why aren't you happy with Daddy?" I asked.

"He's so difficult," she answered flatly. "He doesn't make any money and we fight all the time," she said.

That's true, I thought. My parents often shouted at each other, or my father wouldn't speak to my mother for weeks. Sometimes I'd see her cry, and although that upset me, I learned to take it for granted. It never occurred to me that my family might be torn apart.

"Does Daddy know you're leaving him?"

"He's been playing Go all day in Japantown in San Francisco, so, no, he doesn't know yet. He'll find out when he gets home tonight," she said grimly. Elliot continued to translate for me but otherwise was silent. He watched my face closely to see my reaction to this jolting news.

Poor Daddy, he'll be all alone, I thought. *But maybe Mommy won't cry anymore.*

"Maybe you'll be happier now," I said. I was always concerned for my mother's happiness.

She didn't answer.

"If he makes no money, how'll we live?" I asked her. I was scared. I draped myself over the front seat, trying to hear my mother's answer above the freeway noise.

"I just got a job with Traveler's Aid, so I'll be able to make enough money to pay the rent and food for the four of us. I waited until I got a good job, so now I think I can support us all. I hope your daddy will give me some child support money for the two of you, but I doubt that he will. He hasn't paid the mortgage on our house or property taxes for years, so we owe the bank and the IRS a lot of money. That's why the bank is taking our house away."

We'd left the freeway and were driving through the familiar streets of Berkeley. My heart contracted in an icy grip.

"What about Daddy? Will Daddy still live in our house?"

"We have to sell the house soon to pay off the bank, and Daddy will have to find a smaller place to live," she told us. I was relieved that Elliot and I were going to live with our mother; she was so much more stable and responsible than our father. But I was already missing him. I felt numb, but my mind whirled with practical matters.

"Where's the new house?" I asked.

"It's on Scenic Avenue, just a few blocks from your school. You'll be able to continue going to Hillside school."

"How'll we find our way to school tomorrow?"

"There's a girl, Emily, who lives right next door. She's a year older than you, Claudia. I've already talked with her mother. Emily will walk you and Elliot to school early tomorrow morning after I leave for work. Omama will make you breakfast."

"What's the phone number of the new house, and how'll Daddy find us?" I asked. I was afraid I might never see him again. The conversation was going slowly as Elliot continued to repeat everything our mother said. But I was determined to get the answers to all my questions.

My foundation was crumbling, and I felt I had to take care of these practical matters to keep my world from imploding further. I didn't know how else to do this apart from getting all the details of our new home. My heart sliced in half as my loyalty to my father was split—maybe his instability would no longer loom over our household, and part of me was relieved. But I felt guilty for having these thoughts and I knew I would miss him terribly. I also wanted to be as mature as possible to avoid further upsetting my mother. This continued my pattern where I tried to protect her from my pain so as not to distress her. I was growing up fast.

"I'll give him our new address, and you can visit him sometimes."

She told us the phone number and address of the new house, but I couldn't decipher all her words. Elliot turned to me and clearly repeated the numbers, several times, and I spent the rest of the car ride memorizing the information. When we arrived at the small rental house on Scenic Avenue, my mother pointed out my room. I ran straight past the boxes stacked in the hallway and into my new bedroom where all my dolls and stuffed animals were lined up along my freshly made bed. I flung myself on the bed, swept my dolls into my arms in a big embrace, and cried with happiness to see that my treasured possessions had been transferred to this new home. My mother, in the midst of everything she was going through, had made sure our new home was as welcoming as possible.

The next day, as promised, our neighbor Emily knocked on our door and motioned for us to follow her to school. I felt awkward and didn't know what to say to her, and she didn't speak to us either. But I also welcomed the silence because I couldn't explain that my parents were getting a divorce; I barely knew what the word meant, and I certainly didn't know anybody whose parents were divorced. But somehow it felt shameful.

Elliot and I quickly settled into the new house and life with our mother and Omama, but I was eager to see my father again. Two weeks later, shortly before my ninth birthday, we saw him for the first time since the move. He picked Elliot and me up in a beat-up old black Ford Anglia that he had just bought, as my mother kept the family car. He drove us to dinner at La Val's, the popular Italian restaurant at the bottom of Euclid Avenue in Berkeley near the university campus. Over dinner, with a loud exhale he sighed, "I don't understand. Your mami no longer wants to live with me."

I was surprised at the fury that coursed throughout my body. He wanted our sympathy, but as far as I could see, he was the one who always made our mother unhappy. I was roiling with anger and grief— emotions too complex for me to sort through—and I couldn't speak. I was feeling sorry for him that he was all alone, but I couldn't express my sadness, so I dug into my spaghetti without a word. Elliot didn't speak either, and after dinner our father drove us home in silence.

One Saturday afternoon a couple of weeks later, my mother announced, "Get your sweaters. We're driving over to the LeRoy Street house this afternoon. Daddy and I have to sort through our record collection. You kids can play inside and say goodbye to the house. It's up for sale now."

In the old house, as Elliot and I started upstairs to Elliot's empty bedroom to find something to do, we watched our mother, arms tightly wrapped around her chest, standing awkwardly aside from our father as he pulled LPs out of the record player cabinet and tossed them onto the sofa.

"Wait," our father called out after us. "I found this box of crayons. Take them—the house will be painted next week so you may draw whatever you like on the big wall in Elliot's room." That was my father at his best, showing his willingness to break rules to have fun. I was going to miss his playfulness.

Grabbing the box of crayons, we went up to Elliot's room. We began to draw with determination, me beginning in the lower left corner of the wall, my brother reaching as high as he could to the upper right corner. As I was drawing, I thought about how much I was going to miss our house. Five bedrooms and six baths—I'd always loved counting them. My room littered with stuffed animals and dolls, the walk-in closet where I would cry out my tantrums, and my curtains, printed with cheerful blue and red drums. The labyrinthine basement where Elliot and I played hide-and-seek, scaring ourselves amidst the jumble of old mothballed trunks and boxes. The high swaying branch of the cedar tree I climbed to peer into my father's study. The patch of lawn where my father intended to build a bomb shelter. No longer would this be ours.

We drew with force and fury, with me eventually standing on a chair and my brother now crouched by the floor. I would miss the scent of old-world mustiness of my grandmother's suite down the dark hallway where I used to sit on her bed wrapped in her thick fur throw and watch her select a prim hat with a mesh half veil, which she would fasten on her head with a pearl pin. I loved her potted plant with the tiny heart-shaped leaves that dangled in long strands down to the floor. On a little table near her bed had stood her shrine to grief, photos in silver frames of her relatives she had told me had starved to death in the Theresienstadt concentration camp.

The stately sunken living room with the tall Christmas tree that gleamed in the corner, a radiant queen, adorned with red candles, gold tinsel, and precious wooden ornaments that my mother brought from Germany in her suitcase. The long staircase Elliot and I slid down, riding a regal carriage of blankets, landing tumbled, heaped and breathless below. No longer would this be ours.

But most of all I would miss my father's presence. Although through the years I began to recognize more and more of his flaws, there was so much about him I'd miss. Our reading sessions and cuddles in his study. His affectionate warmth and gigantic bear hugs. His carrying me upstairs over his shoulder and tenderly tucking me in bed after I'd fallen asleep in the living room. The games he taught us and his imaginative playfulness. Although I was told I would see him once a week, I was already feeling the pain of the separation from my father.

An hour later, my father entered the room and turned pale. I stepped back to look and saw with surprise that we had scribbled the wall a solid black.

Chapter Six

After my mother filed for divorce, my father tried to gain full custody of Elliot and me. In those days, custody of children was almost always awarded to their mother, but the custody battle dragged on for three long years as my father, determined to change California's divorce law, repeatedly fired his attorneys and filed new motions. During this time, I was aware of the dispute but neither parent spoke much about it. I mainly knew that my father wasn't paying my mother alimony or child support and that she was anxious about money. She was working hard as a social worker to support us, herself, and Omama, who continued to live with us. My father, she told me, didn't really want to take care of Elliot and me but just wanted to make life hard for her because she'd left him. I winced at the idea that he might not actually want us. But I had witnessed enough of his erratic behaviors, and I'd seen him ignore us enough times to know she was probably right. I was very glad we were living with my mother.

Elliot and I had visits with our father for dinner most Friday evenings, and sometimes we saw him on Sunday mornings. He always took us to La Val's for dinner, where we regularly ordered spaghetti with meatballs. After dinner he drove us downtown for dessert at Edy's, an old-fashioned ice cream parlor. On Sundays we went to Tilden Park for the pony rides, the merry-go-round, and sometimes the children's steam train. If the weather was bad, he drove us to the house he was renting high up on Panoramic Way where we would talk, play chess or dominoes, or work on solving puzzles. Sometimes he read to us, but mostly he regaled us with stories about his patients and his Go tournaments. He asked few questions about us apart from grilling Elliot on his multiplication tables and spelling, which Elliot detested. This arrangement didn't vary for the three years of the custody dispute. It seemed it never occurred to our father to change our routine, and it never occurred to me to ask him to take us to new places.

During this time, I continued to face regular challenges in the classroom because of my hearing disability. Periodically in fourth grade, our class would walk single file down the long wood-paneled hallway to the darkened auditorium to watch nature films of amazing spiders and butterflies that could somehow survive in the desert and flowers that unfurled in slow motion into blazing colors. But there were no lips to read in those films, so I couldn't understand the voice-over narration. Back in class, the discussion about the films were too fast for me to follow. Because I was a dedicated student and a passionate reader, my teachers, busy with classrooms full of students, would simply forget about my disability and the fact that I needed help to follow a class discussion. And my classmates probably just thought I was shy. Nobody seemed to realize I simply didn't understand.

I also experienced painful frustration on Friday afternoons when our teacher would read aloud a chapter from *Charlotte's Web*. She read quickly, and because I couldn't see the words on the page, they burbled meaninglessly over my head, but I steeled myself against the pain of not understanding and pretended to follow the story. During one reading session I saw many of my classmates inexplicably sobbing, some with their heads on their desks. I was mystified. At recess, seeing I was the only girl not crying, the girls formed in a circle around me and asked me something about Charlotte.

"What [*mumble-mumble-mumble*] Charlotte [*mumble-mumble*]?"

I didn't understand, and my face burned; I pretended to be heartbroken, too, and cried. I knew they possessed some truly important

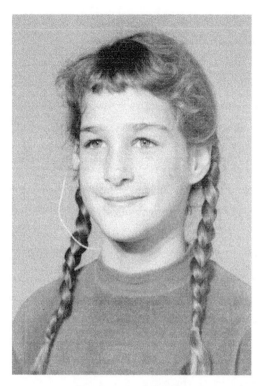

Putting on a brave face

information that I didn't, and my heart constricted in grief. Later that evening I asked my mother to borrow the book from the library, and only after I finished reading the book did I realize that it was when Charlotte, the spider, had died that everyone had cried.

I'd been wearing a hearing aid since I was four, but in the early years—before I started first grade—I'd been content in the quiet of my own world and didn't feel that I was different from other kids. The knowledge that something was wrong with me came to me gradually, starting in early elementary school. At first, I couldn't understand the movies and television that others so easily understood. Then, as I entered the more social years of later elementary school, I noticed I was missing much of what went on between the other kids and in the classroom, and the gulf my hearing loss created in my life at times left me lonely and depressed.

Mostly I tried to ignore my sense of isolation as I knew there was nothing I could do about it, but sometimes the pain of disconnection sliced through my heart. My mother made sure I had as good a hearing aid as possible, that my batteries were fresh, and that the electrical cord connecting the mold in my ear to the hearing aid was changed every six weeks when it wore out. And every new school year, she told my elementary school teacher about my hearing loss to make sure I was assigned a seat in the first row. But beyond that, my parents simply didn't understand how much I struggled to follow discussions in the classroom, in the cafeteria, and in social situations, and I didn't want to create a burden by telling them of my difficulties. My mother, in particular, seemed to have enough problems of her own worrying about money and fighting my father for custody. Adding to my feelings of separateness was the fact that I knew of no one else whose parents were separated or divorced, nor did I know any other kids whose parents were German.

Although I did my best to stay positive despite my ever-increasing sense of not belonging, my father didn't make it easy with his continued bizarre behavior. One afternoon when Elliot and I were visiting him, he asked us out of the blue, "How would you two rascals like to take some LSD?" I was ten, my brother eight, and the three of us were sitting in my father's living room in the house he was renting high above the Berkeley campus. His Go game was arranged on the coffee table littered with Japanese magazines illustrating games played by the masters. I didn't know what to say. I just stared at the Van Gogh book on his coffee table, open to *Starry Night*.

"With LSD you can actually experience your birth again, like my patients do," he told us. *Why would anyone want to experience their birth? Sliding out naked and slimy from between their mother's legs?* I thought to myself and squirmed.

He had told us several times about LSD and his experiences, but never before had he offered it to us. He went on to explain how LSD could be used in psychoanalysis as a tool to uncover very early memories and repressed trauma. But I wasn't interested in uncovering early memories or trauma.

"Will we see wavy curtains, rainbow lights, and shooting stars?" Elliot squealed, spinning in my father's office chair. Our father had described to us some of the visual effects of LSD, and part of me, too, wanted to see walls move, colors radiate, and the world appear in a raindrop, but I continued to sit, silent.

What would our mother think? I wondered. I was distressed that my father would think of giving us something that seemed to be for grownups only.

Several years later I learned from my mother that our father had used LSD with his patients in the '50s and early '60s, well before the widespread use of psychedelics in the late '60s. He was one of the early pioneers.

"Can we do it right now?" my brother asked, legs flailing, spinning the other direction in the chair.

"First, you have to ask your mother for permission," our father said.

What if I remember my birth but forget who I am now? I might get stuck, unable to find my way back to myself.

Mixed with feelings of excitement and anxiety, I couldn't tell him my fears. I desperately hoped my mother would say no.

That afternoon when we arrived home, Elliot rushed to our mother. "Daddy said we had to ask you if we can take some LSD! Pleeease, can we?!"

Flinching, she looked down at us in silence for some time as Elliot went on about what we might experience on LSD. I waited in anticipation to hear what she was going to say.

"Absolutely not!"

She added that if he asked us again, she'd bring up the matter with her divorce attorney. At our next visit Elliot pleaded with our father to give us LSD, but our father said wistfully that our mother forbade it. I was relieved but also disturbed that our father had even considered giving us a substance that our mother could be so adamantly against. Once again, my loyalty was split between my two parents. Loving two people who were so opposed to each other was difficult. I wondered if other children of divorced parents also felt this split in loyalty.

During one of our Friday night visits, Elliot, my father, and I were eating spaghetti in our regular plush red booth at La Val's when our father asked, "Have you rascals ever seen a thousand-dollar bill?" He glanced surreptitiously around the restaurant, then, with a flourish, pulled a bill from his wallet and slapped it down on the table in front of us.

"Rascals, take a close look at this bill, for you may never see one like this again." It was dusk on a hot summer evening, I was wearing shorts, and my thighs were sticking onto the protective plastic covering the leather seats.

"One day when you're older, I'll tell you how I earned this. But for now, it's top secret. Let's call it *Project X*," he said.

I studied the bill in my hands. *What is he doing with this much money? Hadn't our mother told us he wasn't paying child support?* I wondered.

After dinner, as usual, he drove us to Edy's for dessert and allowed us to pick whatever we wanted from the menu. A waitress with a short, frilly pink apron and pointed pink cap took our order. I chose the banana split, and our father flamboyantly insisted the waitress bring me a double helping of hot fudge.

Around this time, he started traveling in the United States for work on *Project X*, but he wouldn't reveal what it was or where he was going. He would write to us via a friend of his who forwarded his letters to us. Because the letters were sent from his friend, the postal cancellation stamp was marked Berkeley, so we never knew where our father actually was. In one letter he wrote:

Dear Rascals, I know you want to know what Project X is, and why it has to be such a secret. But sometimes grown-ups need to keep something a secret in order for it to work out. I know it seems silly, but that's just the way it is. Also, I don't know for sure whether my good idea will actually work—it takes quite a long time to try it out. All I know now is that it looks quite good, and the moment I know, I will come right back to Berkeley. So go on crossing your fingers for the success of the invention because it'd be so nice if I got enough money soon—not only for me to live on (unfortunately, that always has to be paid first, and earned first), but, maybe, maybe, also for the three of us to go away sometime on a trip. How would that be, rascals? And then, if the invention is really good, I could start putting some money aside for the two of you for when you will want to go to college. Let's see.

I have to work very hard for the invention—eight hours a day, and the work is very tiring. More and more I see that there is a part in this invention business that others cannot do as well as I can. So, I am the one that has to do it. On Saturday I'll have my first free day after ten days of work, work, work. You know, a secret is great fun, but more for the person who knows it. But you understand by now that I can't tell anyone. You'd be the first ones to know, of course, if I could tell. Love from your Daddy.

At first Elliot and I were thrilled with the drama of the secrecy, but after a while it became frustrating not knowing what this *Project X* was all about. And I missed not seeing him for six weeks at a time. After a while we stopped hearing about *Project X* and gradually Elliot and I lost interest in it. We didn't know at this time what my mother knew but didn't tell us—that an acquaintance of my mother's had told her that she'd seen my father gambling in Las Vegas. My father had apparently discovered a way of counting cards in blackjack to figure out the statistical odds of certain cards being played, which gave him a slight edge. He'd play patiently for a while in one city, either Reno or Las Vegas, and then, when he made some money—but not so much that he would draw attention to himself—he traveled to the other city to gamble or returned to Berkeley for a time. In this way he was able to systematically make money as this was before blackjack rules were changed to make it impossible to count cards. He was working hard to pay off his mounting debts. Only years later would I learn how much he made, and what he did with the money.

Around this time, one day at school Ellen told me there was a special film the girls were going to watch while the boys were going to go outside and play soccer. Ellen explained that the mothers in the class had all received letters from the school alerting them that "the film" on menstruation was going to be shown. *Oh, so this is what Mommy was trying to tell me about last night,* I thought.

I thought back with embarrassment to our awkward conversation when my mother sat me down on my bed and told me, out of the blue, that soon I would become a woman. I would have to wear a pad in my underpants because I would bleed for a week. This sounded preposterous. I had no idea what she was talking about and instead of asking her any questions, I burst out into a hysterical laughter. My mother, annoyed, said maybe we should talk further about this some other time.

"Have you heard of menstruation?" I asked Ellen, stumbling over the word.

"Yes," Ellen said. "My mother told me about it a while ago, and Lorene started her period two months ago." Ellen told me that was all she, Lorene, and Debbie had been talking about lately.

With a stab of pain, I realized what the girls in my class were probably whispering and giggling about during recess and slumber parties. I watched the film about menstruation, but as usual, I understood little of the voice-over narration. There was a lively class discussion afterwards during which several girls asked questions, but the conversation moved fast, and I couldn't understand the questions or the answers. Once again, I was frustrated not to be part of the discussion but tried to shrug the whole thing off. Stuffing my feelings was a way of not fully feeling the pain of being left out, and as time went on, I used that strategy more and more.

But stuffing my feelings didn't work when I bombed my oral report in fifth grade. My teacher, Kathleen Favors, was the only Black person in an all-white school, and I adored her. I would run to her and beam up at her face when she supervised the playground at recess, and she would lean over and wrap me in a big hug. I didn't see her hug any of the other children, so I felt special. She told us stories about her hard life as a young girl growing up in the South. Attuned to my hearing disability, she often stood in front of my desk while she taught, ensuring I would understand her as much as possible. She enthusiastically told us about the televised Kennedy-Nixon debates; she hoped Kennedy would win the election, so I fervently rooted for Kennedy. I wanted to do well in her class.

Towards the end of the school year, we had to research and write a report on a topic we were interested in. Because Mrs. Favors was Black and had told us with great admiration about how Abraham Lincoln had wanted to end slavery, I decided to do my report on him. I also liked that Lincoln's craggy face and shock of dark hair reminded me a bit of my father.

But along with the report, we also had to give an oral presentation to the class and to our parents. Mrs. Favors required that each student invite a member of the community to hear our presentations. I couldn't think of anyone to ask, so Mrs. Favors suggested I invite

Wilmont Sweeney, a friend of hers, who in 1961 was the first Black person elected to the Berkeley City Council. I knew Mrs. Favors wanted to show me off to Mr. Sweeney, and, because he was her friend, I wanted to do well.

I sensed that he was an important man, and this added to the pressure I was already feeling about speaking in public. I'd always had trouble following class conversations; I hadn't wanted to make a fool of myself by jumping in and unknowingly talking about something different from what was being discussed. As a result, I rarely spoke up in class, and I'd certainly never stood in front of the class to give a report. I was also afraid someone would ask me a question from the back of the room.

On the morning of the presentation when I saw all the parents and guests seated expectantly at the back of the crowded room, I froze with stage fright. I spotted Mr. Sweeney, dressed in a black suit, and my mother next to him, elegant in a navy blue shirtwaist dress. Like a statue I stood at the front of the room, desperately trying to remember what to say as I mumbled my way through the report. Fortunately, there were no questions. I looked over at the audience; Mr. Sweeney had a blank expression on his face, and my mother sat motionless and uncomfortable. My father had told me he couldn't make it to my presentation because he had to compete in San Francisco in an "important Go tournament." I was relieved he wasn't there. But my cheeks burned and I was almost in tears as I returned to my seat; I felt mortified and ashamed of having totally bombed my talk, of having let my teacher and my mother down. But even so, I couldn't bring myself to tell them about my terror of speaking and of being asked questions that I wouldn't be able to hear. Children being taught to advocate for themselves wouldn't come until decades later.

I was too ashamed to confide in my father about my disastrous oral report. Increasingly he had become more and more absorbed in his own world. He rarely asked Elliot or me questions about our lives, our interests, how we were doing in school, or how we were getting along with friends. And he no longer seemed interested in how I was doing with my hearing aid. By not probing to find out how I was faring, he just assumed that I was like everyone else. I didn't want to bother him with my troubles, so I didn't talk to him about my social isolation, my awkwardness, and my embarrassing misunderstandings due to hearing incorrectly.

But during this time my father spent a lot of time teaching us chess and the basic strategies of Go. We were eager to please him and diligently learned the moves. And I liked that he took us seriously and spoke with us as if we were adults. But he often carried on about his preoccupations with the various Freudian theories of psychoanalysis, the teachings of Karl Marx, the actions of the Nazis and the Russians, and Austrian animal behaviorist Konrad Lorenz's theory of human aggression, the fighting instinct that animals and humans have to kill members of their own species. Out of boredom and frustration we'd sometimes compete for our father's attention, squabbling and punching each other, much to his annoyance. I wished he'd occasionally visit us separately to give us each the individual attention we craved and needed, but neither of our parents suggested this.

One afternoon when I was ten, we listened to him pontificate in the living room of his rental house about the Russians and the dangers associated with a possible nuclear attack while Elliot spun around in my father's office chair. Then my father reached over and handed me a book from his coffee table: *Lord of the Flies* by William Golding.

"This is a very important book," he said emphatically. "I want you to read it because you need to learn how humans have the instinct for aggression. This aggression is very dangerous and needs to be controlled."

He was obsessed with this topic and the terrible things humans had done to each other by way of concentration camps, bombing raids, and nuclear attacks, and he believed there needed to be a world government to contain this aggressive instinct. He was particularly taken with Lorenz, who was well known for his work with graylag geese showing that geese, through a process of imprinting, follow the first moving object they see within a few hours after hatching. This, my father said, suggests that attachment is programmed genetically for the survival of the species. I loved the sweet black and white photographs he showed me of the geese following Lorenz around on his farm. But my father was far more interested in Lorenz's work on aggression, and he wanted to engage with him in a correspondence.

"I've sent Mr. Lorenz articles I've written supporting his ideas, but he never writes back. Nobody wants to publish my articles on aggression."

"Why won't anyone publish your articles?" I asked.

"People are very silly. I am working very hard to help form a world government, but people won't listen to me. That's because they don't want to look at the truth about human nature."

I was frustrated by his talk of aggression. This was all far removed from my life, my attempts to fit in at school and to make friends. But at the same time, I was very curious about *Lord of the Flies* because it was about children my age stranded on a remote island. At home that afternoon I read with fascinated horror how, without adults to supervise them, ordinary English schoolboys engaged in acts of cruelty and murder. I wondered whether my classmates and I would, in extreme circumstances, revert to such behavior. *Would we turn on each other? Would we abuse or even kill each other?* And I was struck by the irony at the painful ending when the children were rescued by adults in the middle of fighting a larger war of their own.

The following week, after I had finished *Lord of the Flies*, my father gave me another book, a thin hardcover copy of *Hiroshima* by John Hersey.

"This is another important and grown-up book for you. It'll show you how horrible humans can be with one another. It's very disturbing, so don't let Mami see you reading it. Hide it under your mattress."

I was flattered that he trusted me with this adult book and that I had to keep it a secret from my mother, but I was also scared, knowing that it would be another look into the terrible things people did to each other. I didn't want to read it, but I wanted to please my father. In Hersey's book, published in 1946, six survivors of the atomic bomb share their experience of the August 6, 1945, attack on Hiroshima. Hersey's writing is matter of fact, but I was horrified by his descriptions of how, after the atomic blast, eyeballs were melted and people were vaporized so that sometimes the only trace of them that remained was a shadow of ash imprinted on the walls of the city. I couldn't get these images out of my mind, but I couldn't talk about them with my mother. I knew she'd be angry with my father for giving me the book, and I didn't want to cause more trouble between them. I also couldn't talk about the book with my father. He nodded with approval when I handed it back to him, but he seemed distracted and didn't say a word. By now I wanted to put it all out of my mind and so I didn't ask him any questions.

Ever since his failed venture with the mail order Rorschach test, I'd been losing faith in my father. He was the only person who seemed to see value in his many ideas, and that made me doubt him. I couldn't imagine what he could possibly do that would make much of a difference to world peace. And when he went on about how no one would take him seriously, I couldn't either. So I no longer looked up to him. That made me feel vulnerable and insecure. My father was no longer the solid source of comfort and support he had once been when I was a young child, and the books he had given me made the world seem like a scary place that he couldn't protect me from.

Chapter Seven

I often found solace from my worries in my Brownie meetings on Thursday afternoons. On the shoulders of my uniform, I proudly sewed the badges I'd earned completing the required projects. To earn one of the badges we had to identify and sketch the leaves of the various trees in our neighborhood, and I spent many contented hours at the dining room table completing detailed drawings with colored pencils. For another project, we were taken on a field trip to Lake Anza in Tilden Park where we drew the bugs and beetles we found there. I delighted in these artistic forays into nature. It was beautiful and quiet, and I loved working with the art materials. As I had to rely so much on my visual abilities due to my hearing loss, they were highly developed, and I did well on these projects. I was pleased with my artwork. Even better, everyone was engrossed in their individual projects, so I didn't feel excluded from any group discussions during drawing time.

But the best part of being a Brownie was making gifts for my family. At one meeting shortly before Christmas, we sat around the dining room table of our troop leader's house and were given flat sheets of beeswax that we rolled into candles and decorated with colored sequins and glitter. As sugar cookies baked in the oven, I could faintly hear Christmas carols playing in the background. And, to my happiness, everyone worked in silence, so I wasn't left out of the fast-moving conversation that usually transpired at Brownie meetings.

However, to my dismay, many of the meetings were spent singing songs. In the cacophony of different voices, I couldn't distinguish the words or hear myself sing, so I would just move my lips and mumble along. I was too embarrassed to explain to the troop leader my need to read the lyrics, and she didn't notice my predicament. I tried my best to accept the situation as it was, assuming that there was nothing to be done. The words for many of these songs weren't written out; the girls just seemed to learn them after one recitation by the troop leader, so when it came to singalongs, I was doomed.

Elliot and I continued to be close friends and our shared play often made me forget my father's absence and my hearing difficulties. By now I was a scrappy tomboy and was quite protective of my little brother. Together we engaged in games but also battles with the kids in our neighborhood. One afternoon, as Elliot and I were playing outside, the neighborhood bullies at the end of the street ran up to us and yelled threats. I filled our squirt guns with dishwashing soap, and Elliot and I sprayed the boys who were now completely surrounding us. With soapy water in their eyes, they ran home but soon came back brandishing metal garden spades. Elliot and I dashed into our garage and armed ourselves with metal rakes. Then Ron, two years older than me, pinned Elliot down under him. I picked up a garbage can lid and slammed it down on Ron's head. Ron howled, released Elliott, and ran home. Like a woman warrior I felt a surge of confidence in my ability to protect us.

On other afternoons we tinkered with Elliot's Morse code set, laying down the wire along the hallway between our two bedrooms so we could transmit secret messages to each other at night. We also played games: dominoes, chess, Stratego, Memory, Frisbee, scoop ball, and tennis. My mother had finally bought a television, and Elliot and I were captivated by the surreal plots of *The Twilight Zone* and the action in *77 Sunset Strip*. But I couldn't understand a word that was said on the television. Although I could hear the television's sound, the

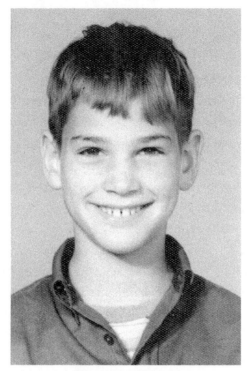

Elliot, eight years old

words weren't clear to me, especially if a show included background music and voice-over narration. In most cases, I couldn't understand the story by lipreading alone, so often, as we cuddled under a blanket on the sofa, Elliot patiently explained what was happening onscreen. In this way he took care of me, drawing us ever closer.

Elliot was also my ears when we were all in the car together. I wasn't able to understand what my mother or other adults said in the front seat as I could neither hear above the traffic noise nor lipread behind their backs, so he would look directly at me and tell me what was going on. When our mother, to our delight, sometimes allowed us to sleep in our sleeping bags on our front lawn on Friday nights, Elliot, ever attuned, shined the flashlight on his face so I could lipread him as he told me jokes. As we gazed at the stars garlanding the sky, he explained to me his understanding of Einstein's theory of relativity, which he'd picked up from our discussions with our father. I was impressed. He was the first of many people I'd rely on over the years to explain the world to me. I was always grateful for the support, but my dependency on others made me feel vulnerable. How would I do without their help?

For our sixth-grade science class project I chose to research and write my report on the human ear. By now I was curious to learn more about my disability, what caused hearing loss, and the history of hearing devices. Determined to do better than I'd done on my oral report on Abraham Lincoln, I wrote a page of notes that I memorized, and I spent many evenings making elaborate colored pencil drawings of the outer, middle, and inner ear to show the class the complex makeup of this important organ. I took special care when I drew the three tiniest bones of the human body—the anvil, hammer, and stirrup in the middle ear—because I was intrigued that my body could have such tiny bones and that something so small could be so vital to our hearing.

The more I researched, the more fascinated I was with the subject. I thought it was miraculous that sound could be produced at all, and I had so many questions. How can these almost transparent bones transmit vibrations from the eardrum to the nerve fibers in the inner ear? How is it that the brain can process these signals to tell between music, speech, and noise? And what is silence but the absence of such signals to the brain?

I also wrote about the dramatic changes in hearing aid technology since its inception. My mother brought me books from the library, and I eagerly plunged into learning about the development of hearing devices, from long ear trumpets to bookshelf-sized contraptions to the type of hearing aid I was now wearing. *I am so glad I wasn't born back in the past,* I thought.[1]

One thing I learned during my research was particularly meaningful to me: why very loud sounds were so difficult for me to tolerate. I learned it was because hearing aid technology didn't yet include the ability to cap the volume of loud noises. That innovation would come decades later with the advent of digital hearing aids. I'd always vigilantly anticipated loud noises so I could spare myself physical pain by turning the volume down on my hearing aid or even turning it off. But often I was taken by excruciating surprise by a loud blast, like when Elliot and his friends fired their cap guns. Ironic as it may seem, extremely loud noises are a real problem for people with severe hearing loss because of the high level of amplification required for their hearing aids.

One of my mother's friends, a doctor, offered to lend me a plastic model of the ear for my presentation. My mother beamed with delight when she brought the model home, unwrapped it from its box, and placed it on the dining room table. But after examining it, I said, "This's definitely *not* an ear." It looked strange to me, not like the diagrams I had studied of the ear's intricate anatomy.

"Where are the three tiny bones, the hammer, anvil, and stirrup?" I asked.

"Here's the ear canal," my mother said. "See how it goes down into the inner ear?" She pointed out how the canal flowed gracefully around into the coiled cochlea of the inner ear. But the model still looked weird.

I insisted again, "I don't know what this is, but I know it's not an ear!"

On the morning of the presentation my mother set the model on the dining room table next to me while I ate my scrambled eggs. To her annoyance, I said, "There's something wrong with this, and I'm not taking it to school."

I trusted my intuition and left the model behind on the table.

When it was time for my presentation, I mustered all my courage and strode to the front of the class. I stuck to my notes, and to my relief I got through my report and nobody asked me any questions. I was satisfied with how I'd done and relieved to have it over.

A few days later my mother told me through bursts of laughter that when she returned the model, the doctor had said, "Oh my God, my nurse gave you the wrong one! This is a model of the female reproductive system!" To my embarrassment, she would go on to tell this story to her friends at parties. But secretly I was pleased I had relied on my certainty and had gotten it right. My self-confidence was growing.

My confidence also grew after I got my report card at the end of sixth grade. On the day of the parent-teacher conference I eagerly awaited my mother's return. She beamed.

"You got a good report card," she said.

My teacher, Mr. Vander Ent, had scrawled on the yellow form: *Claudia is quite the go-getter.*

"What does that mean?" I asked.

"You work hard, and he thinks you're learning a lot from all the books you're reading. I saw your bookworm. It's practically as long as the classroom, and it's by far longer than any of the others."

Our bookworms were made of circular segments of colored construction paper, and we added a segment to our worm on the wall every time we wrote a book report. I was a voracious reader and was proud of my bookworm.

"And, of course, he loves that you're such an excellent soccer player."

Mr. Vander Ent was an avid soccer player from Holland and had introduced the sport to our school.

"Do you think he likes me?"

"Yes, I think he does," my mother said and smiled.

I smiled back.

Soon I witnessed another of my father's painful failures, one that would further complicate my feelings towards him. One Sunday he picked me up for a visit and pointed to a box in the back seat of the car. Elliot was playing with a friend that day, so this was one of the rare times I had my father to myself.

"I'm giving a concert, and we need to staple these publicity photographs onto telephone poles all around Berkeley," he said. I reached back, pried opened the box, and peered inside. It contained fliers with black and white portraits of my father. The photograph was a head-shot taken from a low angle which made him look quite imposing. His wavy black hair and serious expression gave the flier a dramatic feel. Under his headshot the text read: *Concert: Walter Marseille— Schubert's "Winterreise" for Baritone, Saturday at 8 p.m., February 18, 1961, Florence Schwimley Little Theater.*

After taking singing lessons sporadically throughout his life, he was now at age sixty going to give his first serious recital as a Lieder singer. For years, Elliot and I had heard him practice his singing, but even as a hard of hearing child I could hear how forced and tight his voice sounded. And I could see how strained he looked when he sang. So, while I was caught up in his excitement about the upcoming recital, which he said would make him famous, I was also anxious about how he'd be received; would this fail as had his mail order Rorschach test and his attempts at getting articles published?

Judd, one of my father's few friends, drove Elliot and me to the theater which my father had rented for his recital, and the three of us sat in the second row, quiet and expectant. The theater could seat six-hundred people, and just before it was time for my father to take the stage, I glanced in all directions hoping to see a full house. To my dismay I saw only a handful of people sprinkled throughout the audience. As the accompanist, formal in a tuxedo, busied himself at the piano, the room fell silent. My brother scissored his legs back and forth and I rested my hand on his legs to stop him.

At last my father emerged from the side of the stage, stumping ponderously to the piano, then resting his arm on its edge. There was a lukewarm applause. I waited, anticipating his opening line: "A stranger I arrived, a stranger I depart." He was singing the gorgeous but notoriously difficult "Winterreise" (Winter's Journey) by Schubert, which is comprised of twenty-four songs mostly all written in sad, minor keys. The songs—which take almost an hour to sing—tell the story of a lonely traveler who wanders out into the snow on a journey to rid himself of the pain of a lost love. The songs depict the traveler's tumultuous emotions ranging from great to even greater despair. I had heard my father practice the piece in rehearsals at home, and by now I knew it well.

When he sang the first notes, I heard the strain in his voice, and my heart plummeted. With my perfect pitch I could hear he was singing flat, not in tune with the pianist. My brother started swinging his legs again, and this time I pressed my hand hard down on his knee. When he looked up at me, I'm sure he saw the anxiety written on my face. The audience shifted restlessly and coughed, and I watched, now almost frantic, as a few people slipped quietly out of the auditorium. I was thoroughly miserable and would have given anything to be anywhere else.

At the end few people clapped. Judd led us backstage to see my father, who looked gray and exhausted. I was mortified to see that no one else had come to greet and congratulate him. He and Judd exchanged a few words which I couldn't hear. I was desperate to leave. Judd drove me and Elliot home in silence. When our mother met us at the front door I insisted to her, "The crowd gave him a standing ovation!" She looked at me with a blank expression. I knew she had sent a friend to attend the concert and report back to her, so she knew I wasn't telling the truth. But she let it go, neither of us acknowledging what a disaster it had been. Again, I was having difficulty reconciling his failures with the parent I loved.

By the time I was eleven, my parents had been battling for three years through an acrimonious divorce. The custody battle dragged on only because of my father's unwavering belief that he could change California's custody laws. Once, when I was eleven and rifling through my mother's desk looking for a postage stamp, I found some newspaper clippings my mother had saved. One paper reported that my father had told the judge he couldn't pay child support because he had too many "essential personal expenses." Another article read, "German psychoanalyst tells judge he cannot pay child support because he takes singing lessons three times a week." The article went on to report that he wanted to be an opera singer and had been taking singing lessons for thirty years and also that he was taking tennis lessons. He'd also said he couldn't work regularly because he was busy playing in Go tournaments in San Francisco.

I was embarrassed by these accounts of him. And, although I was flattered he wanted custody of us, I was glad I wasn't living with my father. By now I was thoroughly uncomfortable with his obsessions, moodiness, and erratic behavior, and I didn't want to hear more about how the Russians were going to bomb us. I also didn't understand why he couldn't work like other fathers and pay my mother much needed child support. I felt that Elliot and I weren't important to him, certainly not as important as his dreams of becoming famous by singing or playing Go.

Through the three long years of fighting, my father had gone through multiple lawyers. Again and again, he fired his attorneys because they failed in their attempts to gain him custody of us. When my mother finally was awarded custody, my father's last attorney crossed the courtroom, clasped my mother's hand in his, and said, "I want to offer you my sincere congratulations." I cringed when my mother told me this; my father had been so obnoxious that his own attorney wanted to see him lose.

Not long after the trial, my father launched another grenade into our lives. One afternoon in sixth grade while my class was diagramming sentences, I was summoned to report to the office of Mr. Blitz, our principal. As I walked down the dark hallway, I couldn't imagine what I'd done that called for a trip to the principal's office. Then, through the glass panes in the office door, I glimpsed Elliot fidgeting in a chair. As I entered the office, I saw Mr. Blitz and his secretary, seated at their desks nearby, warily watching my father as he paced back and forth across the room. I knew they'd had strict instructions from my mother never to let our father take us off the school grounds as she was afraid he might one day abduct us and take us to Germany where he, and we, would be beyond the reach of American law.

As I stood by the office door my father announced, "I've lost the custody battle, so I'm moving to Munich to start a new life. There's nothing left for me here in Berkeley." Formal and distant in his black wool suit, he looked at his watch and continued, "I have to leave now to catch my plane. I've come to say goodbye. Munich is very far away, so I don't know when I will see you two again."

My body went cold and rigid. I couldn't speak. *Nothing left for him here? What about his two children? Aren't we a reason to stay?* A familiar swamp of sorrow seeped down into my stomach. At the same time, I felt a painful and conflicted aversion towards my father. Why did he have to make his announcement in public and say goodbye to us in the principal's office? I stared down at the floor, mentally tracing the pattern of grain across the wood. Stiff and embarrassed, I didn't want to hug him in front of the observant eyes of the secretary and Mr. Blitz, but he leaned down, gave Elliot and me quick hugs, and then whirled about and abruptly left the room.

I had no idea that I wouldn't see my father again for another three and a half years.

Chapter Eight

I smiled broadly back at my reflection in the mirror. It was the summer just before middle school, I was eleven years old, and my mother had finally allowed me to have my hair cut short. We'd struggled over her desire to keep me in braids; she wanted me to look like a sweet Bavarian girl. But I wanted short hair that would cover the conspicuous knob that connected my hearing aid to my ear. Along with short hair, I would no longer don those Alpine dirndl dresses with aprons my mother sometimes made me wear. I was done with all things Bavarian.

I inspected my ears carefully, turning my head from side to side. The thick electrical cord snaking along my neck to the hearing aid clipped to my undershirt still showed, but I thought my appearance much improved. Soft waves of light brown hair gently framed my face, and my green eyes underneath my dark brown eyebrows shone brightly back at me. I grinned. I looked older, more angular, more grown-up. Maybe I really was ready for middle school.

Then came a bigger change. Soon after my new haircut, my mother received new behind-the-ear hearing aids for me through the California Society for Crippled Children. Now, for the first time, instead of one hearing aid I would have two, one behind each ear. Hearing through two hearing aids at once meant that I'd not only experience increased volume, but I'd be better able to locate the direction sound was coming from, and hopefully, better able to discriminate speech from background noise. These new aids were a thrilling development for me.[1]

That summer I discovered Beethoven. In the evenings my mother played records of his piano sonatas, and I lay on the floor with my head near the speaker, completely transfixed. I read a biography of his life written for adolescents, and I grieved for him. What suffering and fear he must have experienced when, at the age of twenty-six, he began to realize that his hearing was failing. No longer able to hear, he composed his later transcendent works based on his memory of sound, not from actual sounds themselves, which I found fascinating. I also learned that he became increasingly remote as his hearing loss progressed— something I understood all too well. I read his famous Heilegenstadt Testament letter to his brothers in which he describes his anguish at losing his hearing and the resulting isolation, and oh, how I could relate:

> *Though born with a fiery, active temperament, even susceptible to the diversions of society, I was soon compelled to isolate myself, to live alone. If at times I tried to forget all this, oh how harshly was I flung back by the double sad experience of my bad hearing. Yet it was impossible for me to say to people "Speak louder, shout for I am deaf." Ah how could I possibly admit an infirmity in the one sense which ought to be more perfect in me than others, a sense which I once possessed in the highest perfection such as few in my profession enjoy or ever have enjoyed.*

I understood how such isolation could invade a life, and the idea of it scared me. I wondered what my life would have been like if I'd been born before hearing aids were invented. Without hearing aids I was functionally deaf, and I knew that if I'd been born even thirty years earlier, I wouldn't have been afforded the quality of life I was experiencing. So, despite often being frustrated, embarrassed, and lonely, I was still grateful.

I didn't know any deaf people, although I knew that California had a school for the deaf and the blind near the University of California campus not far from my home. My parents chose to mainstream me at public schools rather than send me to the School for the Deaf. My excellent skill at lipreading supplemented the help my hearing aids provided; my hearing loss wasn't severe enough to require that I rely solely on sign language. But this meant I never met any deaf or hard of hearing children, and I fantasized about someday meeting someone like me who could understand what it was like navigating between the deaf and hearing worlds.

My father had anticipated the development of behind-the-ear aids for some years. From Germany he wrote that having sound come into both ears—in effect giving me stereoscopic hearing, allowing me to tell where a sound came from—would make my life easier. He insisted I get them as soon as they became available, but my mother had made no secret of the fact that he'd paid no child support for several years and had no intention of helping her pay for the aids. I hated that I was dependent on receiving these new hearing aids from a charity rather than from my parents. And the name *Crippled Children's Society* made me feel ashamed and defective. More politically correct and less judgmental terms like hard of hearing were still a long way off.

On my first day at Garfield Junior High, away from the relatively secure cocoon of my elementary school, I was in for a shock. Instead of having to get used to just one classroom of new kids, I now attended seven different classes a day. My junior high was packed with preteens from all over Berkeley, and I entered school with no friends, as my two best friends from elementary school had moved away during the summer. In addition, I missed my father. Although I often found his presence oppressive, I also deeply missed Elliot's and my visits with him, his warmth toward me, and his melancholic love that made me feel I was special to him.

Now without a friend by my side to guide me, I was alone and disoriented as I walked through the noisy maze of hallways, lockers, and unfamiliar classrooms and teachers. In addition, my new hearing aids made things worse by overwhelming me with the sheer volume of sound entering my ears. The ever-present cacophony of noise came from all directions. I was subjected to chatter and rustling papers in the classrooms, yelling and slamming lockers in the hallways, and clanking dishes in the cafeteria.

At home I was assaulted by the television, my mother's phone calls, slamming doors, the sharp clack of pots and silverware in the kitchen sink. And as there was yet no cap on the volume built into these aids, loud noises were excruciating. I hated my new hearing aids.

In school, I struggled to separate someone's voice from a noisy background, which made it hard for me to follow conversations as I walked down the school hallway with other kids or to hear over the din of shouting in the cafeteria. Every sound received the same boost in volume from my hearing aids, and because I'd never before heard so much sound at once, I hadn't yet developed the ability to discriminate and focus on important sounds while blocking out others—a simple skill for normal hearing people. I needed people to look directly at me so I could lipread and sort out what I was hearing. Although having two aids made it easier to locate a speaker's voice, I couldn't keep up with the pace of conversations. By the time I found and turned towards the speaker, the repartee would have jumped to someone else, and once again I'd be lost.

Having hearing aids that were hidden beneath my hair turned out to be a mixed blessing. I was now in a new school with kids who didn't know me, so unlike in elementary school where it was obvious I wore a hearing aid as my braids didn't hide them, in middle school the kids had no idea. Not wanting to seem different from the others or to incite pity, I was too bashful and ashamed to tell other people that I needed them to look at me when they spoke. During lunch I'd force myself to join a group of kids sitting at long benches at a cafeteria table, but because I couldn't see everyone's faces, I simply couldn't follow the back-and-forth of multiple free-flowing conversations.

During the first week of school, I spotted a few sympathetic-looking seventh graders and one day I felt brave enough to sit with them during lunch. As soon as I sat down, a girl named Sharon asked, "Did you watch the [*mumble-mumble-mumble-mumble*] last night?"

"What?" I said.

"Did you watch the [*mumble-mumble-mumble-mumble*]?"

"What?" I said again.

"You know, the [*mumble-mumble-mumble*]?" Sharon repeated, looking a bit frustrated.

"Oh yeah, that." I answered with a smile.

"What did you [*mumble-mumble*]?"

My shoulders hunched and my cheeks burned because I had absolutely no idea what she was talking about. I realized that I was now in a precarious situation. Everyone at the table grew quiet, watching to see how I'd respond. I tried to glean from their faces whether I should answer in a happy or sad way, whether to say I liked the mystery subject or not. Since they were looking serious, I decided to say, "Oh, I really liked it; but it was very sad. What'd you think?" I saw right away from their guffaws and bewildered looks that I'd given the wrong answer. Sharon dropped the subject and turned to speak with the girl sitting to her left. Humiliated, I felt the familiar stab of pain in my heart at appearing foolish and at being left out.

I wasn't particularly shy, but other kids must have assumed I was. I was frustrated at being seen as "out of it" or worse, a bit slow. Although I'd started realizing in elementary school that I was different, the price for that difference was becoming increasingly clear: I was slipping away, skidding along the margins of adolescent life, unable to gain traction in a social group. I was growing more self-conscious of my hearing loss.

The negative impact my hearing loss had on my relationship to music and television shows was particularly painful at that time in my life. I couldn't understand the words to the songs playing on the transistor radios that so many kids carried around, so I simply didn't listen to popular music. I couldn't follow the animated conversations my classmates were having about their favorite bands and singers. Likewise, I didn't know much about the television programs everyone was talking about. My mother didn't allow us to watch much television, but this didn't bother me, as I couldn't understand the programs anyway unless Elliot was there to explain what was happening. Hearing aids allowed me to actually hear the TV shows but separating speech from the background music or voice-over narration continued to make comprehension impossible.

But I was determined to try to fit in. I learned to do a fake laugh when the group erupted in a roar of laughter, and I carefully watched faces to read when the laughter would come or whether the conversation had suddenly turned more serious, in which case I was careful not to smile or laugh. Although I didn't want to reveal the extent of my ignorance, inside I cringed at my inauthenticity. If I'd ask the person next to me what the punch line of the joke was, they'd whisper into my ear. But I couldn't hear whispers, and I couldn't lipread if they spoke directly into my ear. One time, a girl I was trying to befriend cupped her hands around my ear to whisper, and her hands on my hearing aid set off the feedback screech. To my dismay, she shrank back in shock. I hadn't been taught how to explain that I wore hearing aids and that it was OK to need and ask for help. I quickly realized that it was simply easier not to ask.

My inability to mix naturally in a group, my fake laugh, and my inability to explain what was really going on with me compounded my feelings of invisibility. I ended up making friends with quiet, introverted, studious kids who were also outside of the popular orbit. I could talk with a friend, one-on-one, if we were facing each other and in quiet settings. I was a good and attentive listener and asked my new friends questions about themselves, which they liked. I learned a lot through these conversations about what was going on, what my classmates were preoccupied with; these friends unwittingly served as conduits to the larger social fabric of school. In this way I would also skillfully find out about my homework assignments.

"Leslie, what're you gonna do your history report on?" I asked one friend after I'd walked out of class clueless about what the homework was or when it was due. "Do you think you'll be able to get it done by the time it's due?"

"I dunno. Mr. Peterson said we could do it on anything we want as long as it's about the early settlements in America. I'm gonna do mine on the Salem Witch trials, but maybe I'll do it on the Pilgrims' colony at Jamestown. Or Plymouth. My mom says we're descended from the Mayflower, so maybe I'll do it about the Mayflower."

She went on to complain that two weeks wasn't a lot of time for a first draft, especially because of the set of algebra problems due the following Friday. This kind of response offered a goldmine of information.

Then there were the seating charts. On the first day of seventh grade, as we filed into algebra class, our teacher immediately assigned us alphabetically to our seats according to our last name. "M" fell in the last row, and I was placed in the back of the room. This was just awful, but I didn't speak up. As the day went on, every teacher assigned our seats in the same way, so I was seated in different locations throughout the various rooms, but almost never in the front where I really needed to be. We moved from class to class and the teachers had no idea I was hard of hearing. If I happened to be designated to the front row, I was able to hear and follow the teacher and I would get an "A" in the class. But if I was assigned a seat in the middle or back of the class, I'd struggle to follow what was going on, and my grade would suffer. Math was a particular problem because the teacher turned his back to the class to write equations on the blackboard, which made it impossible for me to lipread. Not wanting to draw attention to myself and too ashamed to explain my predicament to my teachers, I felt helpless. And I wanted to protect my mother from my struggles, so I didn't tell her what I was going through. Now, in the wilds of junior high, I was on my own.

No matter where I sat, though, I rarely participated in group discussions; they would go by too rapidly to follow and lipread. Occasionally a teacher asked for my opinions about whatever we were discussing, and several times I earnestly replied to what I thought the topic was, only to see the teacher looking nonplussed and the students sniggering.

But I desperately wanted to fit in and to be seen. Once, when we were learning about the Civil War in my history class, I stayed up late and studied the segment in the textbook thoroughly. The next day, when Miss Wilson called on me, I plunged in, giving an elaborate and enthusiastic monologue about the attack on Fort Sumter that started the Civil War, not realizing that the discussion had shifted to the Reconstruction Act of 1867. The class went silent, the kids gawked at me, and Miss Wilson looked confused. After that I avoided making eye contact with my teachers so I wouldn't get called on, and when I *was* called on, I said, "I don't know" even if I thought I had an answer.

One evening, after my mother cheerfully asked how school was going, I broke down and sobbed and told her about my frustration about the seating charts. She was adamant that it was time for me to take matters into my own hands.

"You need to take care of this yourself. Tell each teacher the first day at the beginning of each semester that you're hard of hearing and that you need to sit in the front row."

I knew she was trying to empower me, but I didn't know how to tell my mother that I was completely frozen, unable to speak to the teachers. I wanted the teachers to know my situation, but I simply didn't have the skills or maturity to tell them myself. My mother couldn't understand my mortification and paralysis and remained insistent I handle things myself. I couldn't share with her the details of my quiet suffering, nor did she ask me to explain more. I knew it was important to her that I be as normal as possible, so we had an unspoken agreement that I was doing just fine.

After a while, I no longer spoke to her about the seating charts or the demerits I was earning because of my lack of class participation because I knew she'd tell me to take care of it myself. It would have been an easy solution for my mother to talk to the school counselors at the beginning of each semester and ask them to draft a note to my teachers, telling them why I needed to sit in the front row. I wished she would have, but she couldn't or wouldn't acknowledge to either of us that I still needed her support.

I felt I was an anomaly, trying hard to "pass" in a hearing world. Often, I was on the outskirts, painfully isolated and disconnected. I was hampered not only by my physiological disadvantage and the limitations of hearing aid technology but also by my unwillingness to call attention to myself. To make it all worse, this was the '50s and early '60s when girls weren't taught to be assertive or to advocate for themselves. I didn't speak up, didn't admit the truth of the hearing loss I believed would make people think I was broken in some way. Speaking up for myself would come years later. Until then, I learned to fake and hide.

Then one day something wonderful happened: I found a best friend. As I was leaving my art class, the girl who for weeks had been sitting quietly next to me asked, "Do you want to walk to PE together?"

"Oh yes!" I answered, thrilled.

We fell into an easy conversation about our classes, what we thought about our teachers, and about the big upcoming art project. Her name was Kirstin, and to my extreme delight we became virtually inseparable, spending most afternoons in the backyard of her house near the school. The first things I noticed about Kirstin were her full red lips, her sky-blue eyes, and the corners of her mouth, which turned upwards into what looked like a permanent smile.

Her honey-colored hair fell loosely in shoulder-length ringlets, and I saw she was already developing breasts. She was round, soft, and pink—everything I, angular and sharp, wasn't. Even her handwriting was round, with little circles in place of the dots of i's. She was sunny, bubbly, and popular, and she wanted to be with me!

It wasn't long before Kirstin noticed my hearing aids. She was fascinated and wanted to know everything about my hearing loss. I told her some things about it, but I was too shy to reveal to her how difficult it made my life. But she quickly learned to speak clearly, always looking straight at me, and she understood that I needed some things explained, like that for our drawing project we could use only charcoal and that we had to concentrate on the shading of light and dark. She became my lifeline. Thanks to this new friendship I began to relax and looked forward to going to school.

I was also slowly getting accustomed to my new hearing aids. The increased volume was no longer quite so overwhelming, and I was hearing things I'd never heard before, like the kids talking behind me in class. Still, without lipreading I couldn't understand what they were saying. The biggest joy I gained thanks to my new hearing aids came by way of improved resonance of piano notes, which were easier for me to discern than people's words; they were clearer, richer, and better defined, so I truly looked forward to my daily piano practice. At this point, I'd been studying the piano passionately for five years, and my mother was very encouraging of my playing, often releasing me from chores so I could practice. And it didn't hurt that Kirstin was intrigued when I showed off the Mozart sonatas I was working on when she came to spend the afternoon at my house.

Before I started junior high, my mother had the idea that I should join the school orchestra. She thought it might help me meet some nice musical kids. But as the orchestra already had a pianist, the conductor suggested I learn the double bass over the summer. The school lent me an instrument, and the conductor gave me a few lessons. By the fall, she said, I'd be able to join the other three bass players in the orchestra. Practicing in my room, I felt the vibrating wooden body of the bass against my torso, its dark pitches streaming from the scrumptious traction of my bow against the strings. But when the school rehearsals started, I couldn't even begin to distinguish the low notes of my bass from the blare of the horn players in front of me and the drums pounding behind me, nor could I orient myself by listening to the other three bass players; I simply couldn't hear them over the cacophony of sound. I played along the best I could, but I'd quickly lose my place.

After our first school concert, Kirstin said, "You know, you were bowing in the opposite direction and were using completely different fingering from the other bass players. Don't you know your part?" I winced as she pointed this out, chagrined at how obvious it had been to my best friend that I'd been completely lost. That evening when my mother asked, "How'd the concert go?" I avoided answering her and said that I was too busy between piano practice and schoolwork and that I needed to quit the orchestra. I didn't want to explain my inability to hear the bass, as I knew we'd both have to acknowledge how much my hearing loss was affecting my life. I preferred she be disappointed in my quitting because of schoolwork than learn the extent of my hearing struggles. In my way, I was again protecting my mother, not wanting her to witness my difficulties and pain. She had gone through so much herself—growing up in Nazi Germany, her difficult relationship with my father, and supporting us as a single mother. Out of love for her I wanted to be strong and confident. I just wanted her to be happy. But my mother and I were paying a price for our mutual silence; by not acknowledging my difficulties, we couldn't be completely authentic with each other.

Kirstin and I were just twelve years old and gloriously in love. Beneath a floral sheet we draped over a dwarf cherry tree in her backyard, we hunched cross-legged, our heads touching, perfecting a sign language alphabet we spent hours inventing. I initiated this activity after having recently witnessed a deaf couple signing to each other on the sidewalk. I'd been completely mesmerized by the beauty and ease of their gestures and was inspired to make up signs Kirstin and I could use. During tests at school we finger spelled answers to each other, our hands discreet beneath our desks. I loved that we didn't have to speak, that I didn't have to hear to understand.

In addition to hours spent practicing our sign language, we explored our neighborhoods, clambering over trashcans and wire fences into backyards to spy on people. Other afternoons we spent at Codornices park near my house on the slides and swings before returning home to huddle together over our homework. Always grateful, I relied on her guidance as to what was expected of us in our assignments. In the Berkeley Rose Garden, we collected petals to press into heart-shaped photo albums we made for each other. One radiant afternoon we pricked our fingers with a thorn and mixed our blood, then cut locks of our hair and tied them with a thin red satin ribbon. We became inseparable. Our close bond made me forget my hearing struggles and for a while I felt normal.

I thought this happiness would last forever. We were too timid to kiss each other, but during an overnight at her house, we zipped our sleeping bags together, and in our pajamas we wrapped our arms around each other. We finger spelled back and forth to each other what we dared not speak aloud: "Maybe this summer at camp we'll kiss each other."

Then *it* happened. At camp we were assigned to different cabins, and she became best friends with Theresa. One morning, we crossed paths as she walked with her arm around her new friend's waist. Kirstin, smiling as always, didn't look at me and just kept on walking. My heart turned to ash. I was once again alone.

That fall, back in school, she started hanging out with more popular girls, and a boy with slicked-back hair. I couldn't bear to see her and went out of my way to avoid her. We never spoke again.

Chapter Nine

As I entered eighth grade, once again I started the school year without a friend. I was relieved to discover that Kirstin wasn't in any of my classes, but sometimes I noticed her in the hallway chatting gaily with her new friends. At lunchtime I sat as far away from her circle as possible.

Kids clustered together in noisy gatherings, and sometimes I sat nearby and tried to follow the rapid conversations, but I couldn't understand enough to interject a comment. And with no one to explain what everyone was talking about, I drifted, invisible, through the long days as the warm Indian summer turned into a golden California autumn. The beauty of the light and the turning leaves made my isolation and loneliness even more painful. *I shouldn't be this unhappy*, I thought, *everyone else looks cheerful; this's just not normal.* The social isolation plunged me into a leaden, sluggish depression.

During those first few weeks of school I cried myself to sleep at night, and I told my mother I didn't want to go to school because I had no friends. I still couldn't explain to her how hard it was to insert myself in social situations. But she was sympathetic to my unhappiness and one evening said, "By Halloween you'll make a friend, I promise you." That night I felt comforted by her words, but by the gray dawn of morning I knew there was nothing she could do to help me connect with others; I had to face another day alone. I dressed in slow motion and dragged my feet down the hill to school.

One day in mid-October as I left the cafeteria with my tray of sloppy joes and canned spinach, I looked around for somewhere to sit and spotted a thin girl with a thick, glossy brown braid that fell all the way to her waist. She was eating at the end of a noisy table and since there wasn't an empty seat near her, I didn't approach her. But over the next few days it seemed I saw her wherever I turned—in the hall, between classes, and out on the soccer field. I thought it strange that she seemed to change her clothes in the middle of the day; sometimes I saw her wearing a dress in the morning and then a completely different outfit in the afternoon. But she always wore the same thick braid down her back. Someone told me her mother was of Ukrainian descent and her father English and that she had been in school in Switzerland for the past year, so she didn't know anyone at our school. I thought in this way she was like me—maybe she also didn't feel at home in her new school. All this made her seem exotic.

Then one day in the hallway I thought I was seeing double. I saw *two* of them talking together, and as I drew closer, I realized that there was more than one braided girl. They were identical twins! They didn't have lunch at the same period, so there was only one of them in the cafeteria during my lunchtime. The next day I walked to where the one braided girl was sitting and asked her name. "Neila," she said. She scooted over, motioned for me to sit down, and after a brief conversation she shyly asked, "Do you want to walk home with me after school?"

My world exploded into a million golden suns.

Soon I met Neila's twin, Lynne, and we discovered that we lived only four blocks from each other. My mother was right; but not only had I made a new friend by Halloween, I had two new friends! I grew to love them both, and soon we were spending most afternoons together at one or the other of our homes. They got along splendidly with each other and had no trouble sharing me between them. Although we didn't share any classes, Neila and I had lunch together every day, huddled against each other deep in endless conversation. For Halloween the three of us dressed up as gypsies from clothes we fashioned together from our mothers' closets and went trick-or-treating together, arm in arm. As my friendship with the twins developed, my depression dissipated, and I looked forward to school every morning. I suspected they gravitated towards me because they, too, lived in a world of their own and noticed a kindred spirit.

Although we were almost thirteen, we played the imaginative games typical of younger children. We dug out a fort under the deck along the front of my house and lined the fort's wooden walls with postcards of Munich, Paris, and London, all places we wanted to visit when we got older. Scrunched together in our subterranean fort we swapped secrets, complained about our strict European mothers, and talked about our teachers and school. I showed them my hearing aids, but even though I felt connected to them it was still too painful to tell them of my periodic loneliness and difficulty making new friends, a truth that was hard to admit even to myself. I did explain, though, how it was hard to follow the teachers' lectures and how math class was particularly difficult because the teacher would turn his back and talk while writing on the blackboard. I was pleased as they asked me lots of questions about what I could or could not hear.

As with past friends, I learned about the adolescent dynamics of our classmates by catching snippets of the twins' gossip. They went out of their way to fill me in and actively sought out interesting tidbits to impart to me. And as I'd developed with Elliot so long before, these connections with friends were vital as they helped make sense of the world around me. I didn't feel so left out when they filled in details that I was simply not able to hear in the midst of adolescent social dynamics.

"Sherry just got her period; that's why she was absent last week."

"Ben kissed Patty at the dance, and she really likes him. But her parents found out and they won't let her go out with him because they think he's too old. He's a junior at Berkeley High."

I spent a lot of time at their house. But like my mother, the twins' mother was strict, and when she disciplined them, usually for what seemed to me like a minor infraction, the punishment often was that they weren't allowed to play with me. To my pleasant surprise my mother was sympathetic and agreed with me that it wasn't fair, that I shouldn't have been made to suffer as part of the twins' punishment.

Shortly before Christmas, Neila planned for us to go ice-skating downtown at Iceland, Berkeley's ice-skating rink. But the twins had gotten in trouble sassing their mother when she told them one evening to stop making such a racket while doing the dishes. Their punishment was that they couldn't go to Iceland with me. What hurt was that the punishment was focused on me in particular; their mother didn't forbid them from taking the bus and going ice-skating themselves—just not with me. To my delight my mother went along with the twins' idea that I should go separately by bus to Iceland and "accidentally" bump into them there.

On the day of the outing, I took the same bus as the twins but sat slouched down in a seat in the back, so it wouldn't look like we were together. Once at Iceland we spent two hours skating around and around the rink, the three of us holding mittened hands on the ice. I beamed deliriously, soaring around the rink with them in the crisp, cold air to the accompaniment of the piped-in holiday music. Then we repeated the same sneaky process returning home. Their mother never found out. "I am so glad," my mother said, smiling at me, after I regaled her with stories from the afternoon. My heart flew out to her for her support and obvious pleasure in my happiness.

One morning in the middle of my English class, a somber, pale teacher entered the room and strode over to our teacher, Mrs. Johnson, who was sitting at her desk grading papers. He rested his hand on her shoulder and whispered into her ear. She gave out a low moan, there was more whispering between the two of them, and then he quickly left the room. Mrs. Johnson lowered her head to her desk and broke out into sobs. I assumed he had told her some bad news about her family. Then she looked up at us and said something in a quiet voice that I didn't understand. The whole class jerked back with a unified gasp. She asked that we observe a moment of silence. Standing in front of us she lowered her head and closed her eyes. I peeked around the class and noticed the others also had their heads lowered and their eyes closed as well. A few of the girls were crying.

Clearly something momentous had happened. I asked Nora sitting next to me, and she whispered something, but I couldn't make out what she said. Tears of pain and frustration filled my eyes at being left out of what was obviously a crucial event. Mrs. Johnson dismissed the class shortly afterwards, and I went into the hallway where stunned students and teachers milled about aimlessly; I'd never seen grown-ups looking so upset and vulnerable. I was desperate to find someone I could ask what had happened, and the twins were nowhere to be seen. Finally, I bumped into Lorene, whom I knew from elementary school and asked her, "What in the world is going on?"

"Didn't you hear? President Kennedy has been assassinated!"

I didn't know what assassinated meant but it didn't sound good. Before I could ask more, Lorene left to catch up with her friends.

I spent the rest of the day through math and PE anxiously waiting to go home so I could find out more. My mother had returned home from work early and when I arrived, she enfolded me in a big hug. Like the teachers at school, she looked distraught, her face pale.

"What happened to President Kennedy?" I asked.

"He was shot and killed while he was riding in a car with Jackie in Dallas."

"Why?" I asked.

"We don't know yet."

She wanted to invite some of her friends over that evening for an informal memorial and asked me to help her get the house ready.

While she made phone calls, I vacuumed and dusted the living room and put together a vase of red roses I picked from the garden. I found a portrait of President Kennedy from a *Life* magazine lying in a stack on the coffee table and put it into a simple frame. Clearing off the magazines I draped a blue velvet cloth on the table and placed the portrait, flowers, and a candle on top. My mother put her arm around me and murmured her appreciation for my efforts.

When her group of friends came over after dinner, I greeted them at the door as they hugged me and each other. Then they quietly took seats on the sofa and the dining room chairs I had set around the coffee table. My mother gave me a plate of nuts, olives, and crackers to pass around. As I sat with them in the living room, they whispered amongst themselves. One woman wept openly as her husband held her hand. I wished desperately that I could hear what everyone was saying and participate in the conversation too, but they murmured too softly. I consoled myself with the thought that I'd be able to read the details the next day in the newspaper. With frustration I tried to understand what was said on the television during the funeral procession, but I've never forgotten the image of the somber crowd, of Jackie's dark, pale beauty, and little John Jr.'s salute.

At this time, John, a professor at UC Berkeley, had become firmly ensconced in our lives. A few years earlier, when I was six, he was a twenty-one-year-old PhD student at the university and came to see about renting a room in our house on LeRoy Avenue. My father had liked him and chose him over the other candidates because he seemed quiet and might make a good chess partner. John, however, was too busy conducting experiments at the university laboratory to play chess, and later, after my parents separated, John moved to Princeton to finish his PhD thesis. We didn't see him for over a year. Then, at only age twenty-six, John was offered a professorship at UC

Berkeley in the molecular biology department. By then I was ten and my parents' divorce was well underway. Upon his return, John and my mother started spending time together at our house on Scenic Avenue.

Early on when John came to the house for dinners on the weekends, Elliot and I would fling ourselves at him and he would help us climb up his body and stand on his shoulders. After dinner he played Stratego and Memory with us, regaled us with fascinating stories of the Swiss psychologist Piaget's theories about how children gradually grow to perceive and experience the world, and drew elaborate pictures of volcanoes and dinosaurs on my painting easel. On the weekends we splashed with him in the surf at Stinson Beach or we all piled in the car and drove to Mt. Tamalpais to fly kites, hike, and play ball—all things our father had never done with us.

Sometimes John came with his toolbox and fixed things around the house to our mother's great pleasure and relief. When the owners of our house on Scenic Avenue unexpectedly sold the house on short notice, we had to quickly move out. Fortunately, John and my mother soon found a house for us near the Berkeley Rose Garden on which John generously paid the down payment. He wasn't living with us, but we saw him often, and when he was around, my mother was light-hearted in a way I'd never seen. Seeing her like that took a load off my mind. I thought, *now it's his job to make her happy.*

One evening, when I was twelve, I perched on the edge of the bathtub and watched my mother put on makeup as she dressed to go out for dinner with John. As she pursed her lips to apply a deep coral lipstick and turned her head from side to side to examine herself, I asked, "Why don't you and John get married?"

In the mirror I saw her blush.

"Oh, I don't know," she said shyly. "He's twelve years younger than me."

I was disappointed but accepted her answer. I didn't see why that age difference would matter, but I didn't ask any more questions.

Sometimes John came with us on our periodic weekends to Columbia, a small town three hours away in the Gold Country of the Sierra Nevada foothills. My mother's friend Marion Rosen had a little cabin there, which she often let us use. Sometimes we went there with Marion and her daughter Tina, who was two years older than I. Often on Friday evenings after my mother got home from work, we would throw together our sleeping bags, duffel bags with clothes, and two days' worth of groceries and take off in John's silver Peugeot. We always broke up the three-hour drive with dinner at the same 1950s diner in Tracy where we ordered hamburgers and cherry pie à la mode. Saturdays and Sundays we spent on the Stanislaus River baking in the sun on a narrow strip of beach under the Ponderosa pines, toyons, and native oaks. When we got too hot, Elliot and I jumped into the glacier-fed river and swam to the other side with John. Other times, while John and my mother lay on beach towels in the hot sand and talked, read, or napped, Elliot and I would explore upriver with our inner tubes.

I loved these weekends, mainly because my mother was more relaxed with John and Marion around and less strict with Elliot and me, letting us roam the town of Columbia and the river unsupervised. These trips to Columbia and time spent on the river were some of the happiest times of my childhood.

But during this time I thought periodically of my father in Germany. He wrote regularly to Elliot and me about his life in Munich, his various projects, and his lawsuit against the university of Munich for violating students' free speech. I felt an undertow of sadness drag through my body when reading his letters, particularly because of his lack of interest in what was going on in my life, and I was bored of hearing about his day-to-day life in such detail. It felt so different to spend time with John. He paid attention to us and played with us in a way our father never had. Elliot and I loved him.

Chapter Ten

I could ski fast, but Elliot and I could barely come to a stop. The snowplow, all we could manage, was completely ineffective on the icy inclines of the Dodge Ridge Ski Resort in the California Sierras.

It was Christmas vacation shortly before my thirteenth birthday, and by now John was a regular fixture in our lives, visiting us at our house more and more frequently and traveling with us on vacations. That afternoon, my mother and John went off to ski together on the higher, more advanced slopes, and Elliot and I were thrilled to be left unsupervised on the intermediate slopes. As we chased each other down the hills, I gloried in the silky glide of my rental skis scrunching along the powdered snow that covered the ice. At first we followed the First Aid team, enjoying the drama as they lifted casualties onto their sleds, covered them in a yellow tarp, and eased them down the hill. Then Elliot and I decided to take the T-bar up to some higher slopes. We were free, it was a bright, crisp blue day and my heart exploded with joy as we were pulled up the mountain.

The T-bar took us higher than I expected, and as I stepped off, I tumbled down the short incline onto the flat landing area as the T-bar seat almost snapped me in the face. A bit shaken, I hoisted myself up by leaning on my poles, then aimed the tips of my skis straight downhill and stared down the mountain. "Watch out for those rocks over there," I told Elliot. "I'll race you down." Marshalling my courage, I pushed off. The snow gleamed crystalline white on the trees, and away from the motorized noise of the T-bar, all was silent. The only sound I could hear—rather, the vibration I could feel—was the slick swish of my skis on the snow beneath me.

After a time, I glided towards some pine trees at the edge of the slope, and I crouched and ducked my head to avoid the branches flicking into my face. Suddenly, I heard the loud scrape of my skis as I skidded on a patch of ice that had formed under the shade of the trees. I tried to snowplow, but I was going too fast and my legs weren't strong enough to bring me to a halt. Completely out of control I landed on my side with a hard *thud*, then tumbled and bounced down the hill, my skis still attached to my boots. Eventually, after about fifty feet, I gradually came to a stop face down in the snow, my right leg twisted around me at an unnatural angle, the back of the ski pointing skywards. Frantically I checked to see if my hearing aids were still on and felt a rush of relief to feel them still in place. As I lay in the snowbank, I felt strangely woozy, and I guessed from the deep unfamiliar throbbing in my leg that I'd broken a bone. I was thirsty and with my mittened hand, I scraped snow into my mouth. "I think I broke my leg. I think I broke my leg," I mumbled over and over again.

Eventually, a man skidded with a flourish of powdered snow to an abrupt stop next to me. It took him a while to release my skis from my boots, unwind my leg, and flag down the First Aid team. Then I watched in a dreamlike trance as the First Aid team whooshed up to us.

Just as the paramedics eased me onto a sled, Elliot skied by. His jaw dropped when he recognized that it was me being lowered down the hill to the First Aid tent. Without stopping he skied the rest of the way down the hill and managed to track down John and my mother, who were told by the paramedics that I was being taken to the little hospital in Sonora. I was rushed there by ambulance, the sirens blaring all the way.

At the hospital, I was loaded onto a gurney, and John held my hand in the X-ray room as they cut off my boot with a small saw. I clamped my teeth together so I wouldn't cry out in pain as they continued to work on me. I was afraid they might cut into me but before long, my leg was secure in a heavy plaster cast from my foot all the way to the top of my thigh, and the stability of it made me feel better. After I was wheeled into a single room, my mother tiptoed in and pulled up a chair next to me and held my hand. "The X-rays show you have broken your leg in five places," she said. "We need to see a specialist to see what needs to be done next."

The next day I was taken by ambulance to the Kaiser hospital in Oakland, where the orthopedist decided, much to my relief, that if my leg was kept raised horizontally, parallel to the floor, for the next five months while the pieces knit themselves back together, I wouldn't need surgery. But I wouldn't be allowed to stand upright or use crutches to get around and I would have to miss school for the next five months, at least. Worse than the pain in my leg, my heart sank at the thought of being isolated at home alone without being able to see the twins every day. Unlike my peers who spent hours every day talking on the phone with their friends, I could barely hear on the phone. I was afraid I'd lose my vital connection with Neila and Lynne and the world they shared with me.

Despite my fear about being away from school, on my first day home from the hospital I was happy to be in my bedroom again, reunited with my stuffed animals, my collection of Japanese porcelain dolls sent by a pen pal, and my bookshelves filled with novels. Elliot kept me company with card games. My mother rented a wheelchair with a leg extension so my right leg could stick out straight in front of me, as required by the orthopedist. As my mother had to return to work the next day, she hired an elderly woman, Liz, to take care of me during the day. Liz was kind, but she left me alone most of the time apart from bringing in meals and helping me to the bathroom. I could be transferred from the bed to the wheelchair with Liz or my mother holding my leg out straight and then onto the toilet to use the bathroom. I'd no choice but to overcome my shyness about my mother and others witnessing me on the toilet seat.

Omama couldn't help me. She'd been gradually declining, suffering from a series of strokes, and had been recently moved to an assisted living facility. I missed her terribly, but she was like a helpless child at this point, a smile permanently plastered on her face and unable to feed herself. She was no longer the Omama I had known and loved so deeply. Although I had plenty of books to read, I dreaded facing the aloneness of the coming months without her, without my family or any friends to keep me company. I assumed that loneliness was hard for anyone, but I guessed it might be even worse for me as it brought back memories of the times I was isolated on the playground at school, during neighborhood games, and at parties.

That first evening at home, my leg throbbed painfully, so I took some painkillers that the hospital had prescribed for me. Still the pain kept me awake, so my mother gave me one of her sleeping pills. Soon the pain lessened and, eventually, I fell into a deep sleep. But sometime later I jerked awake in abject terror, my heart thundering in my chest and temples. I reached over and switched on the standing lamp by my bed. I couldn't figure out what was happening to me as the walls of the room wavered back and forth, and winged black creatures the size of small dogs circled overhead. They had grimacing, contorted human faces and large webbed, bat-like wings. Some came close to landing on my face, and I thought they were going to smother me. I was afraid I was going crazy.

Part of me knew these black demons couldn't possibly exist, and yet I saw them clearly. How could that be? I tried desperately to focus on the facts: I had a broken leg, I was in my room in my bed, Elliot was sleeping in his bedroom across the hall, and my mother and John were nearby. But my heart was racing so hard I could feel the blood pounding in my ears. It took all my self-control to keep from being swept into the world of the circling monsters. I put on my hearing aids and rang the cowbell that my mother had placed by the side of my bed so I could summon her.

"There are black devils flying around in the room," I cried out as she rushed in. "They want to suffocate me."

Immediately she phoned the Kaiser hospital hotline and then slowly explained to me what they were telling her. "I told the doctor that you'd taken some painkillers and one of my sleeping pills. He said you're having a bad response to the combination of the two drugs."

"How does he know?"

"He looked up the side effects of the drugs, and sure enough, you're having a rare reaction to the combination of the scopolamine in my sleeping pill and your painkiller. It can cause you to panic and to see things that aren't really there."

"Has this happened to other people?" I asked, desperate. "When will it end?"

"It's an uncommon reaction, but it's happened before because it's included in the list of drug interactions. The doctor says you'll feel better in a few hours and that you should just relax, not worry, and try to get some sleep. It'll be over as soon as it works its way through your body." She seemed untroubled, and I tried to take comfort from that.

Soon my mother, John, and Elliot left my room, leaving me alone with the overhead light on. I held on to this seemingly rational explanation of a drug interaction with every ounce of sanity that I could retain, but my visions seemed so real. What if the doctor didn't really know what he was talking about? The room was whirling, and I could barely see beyond the winged demons in front of my eyes. I pressed my fingernails hard into my palms and tried to focus; I was in my bedroom, it was just a bad drug interaction, it would pass. But then the books on my bookshelf began to rock from side to side, flapping their pages. They had talons, which they stretched out before them as they took flight and joined the black bats circling around the overhead light. Cowering under the covers, I spent the rest of the night trying to keep a hold of my mind and not be pulled down by the undertow of a nameless dread. I worked hard to claw my way back to reality.

Finally, as the early morning light filtered through the venetian blinds, I felt calmer and was able to fall asleep. When I woke, my mother had already left for work. Although I felt disoriented and lonely, my terror was gone. Liz brought a tray of cereal and banana for breakfast but didn't say anything about the previous night's events. I figured my mother hadn't told her what happened; after all, it was only Liz's second day on the job.

Later that morning my leg was throbbing badly, and I took a couple of painkillers as prescribed. But there would be no more sleeping pills for me! Liz went back into the kitchen, and I opened Charlotte Bronte's *Jane Eyre* to where I had left off.

Within half an hour my heart started pounding in my chest again, and the bats returned. This episode was even scarier than the one the night before because now I was filled with paranoia about it happening again. My visions *weren't simply* because of two drugs interacting. I was now truly convinced I was going crazy, and I thought the doctor and my mother were lying to me. Feeling my heart race and seeing flying bat creatures as the sun was shining through my window was particularly terrifying. Daytime was the time of reality, not of nightmares.

I desperately wanted to talk to my mother, but the phone with the volume adapter was down a narrow hall that the wheelchair couldn't navigate. I called out to Liz and asked her to phone my mother at work, who reported back after talking to the same doctor that evidently there was still enough scopolamine in my system that the drug interaction had been reactivated when I took the painkillers that morning. My mother told Liz to tell me to wait it out, that the panic and visions would eventually subside. Again, alone in my room, I tried to hold onto the idea of a drug interaction and not get dragged under by my terrified thoughts that this might never end, that I was losing my mind.

From work my mother phoned Herbert Goldstein, a kindly old friend of Omama's, and asked him to visit me that afternoon. He entered my bedroom with a bright smile, his leather-bound collection of the *Original Fairy Tales from the Brothers Grimm* tucked under his arm. He pulled up a chair alongside my bed, and for the rest of the afternoon read his favorite stories, at times holding my hand reassuringly, until my mother returned home from work in the evening. Some of the stories he read were the ones our grandmother had read and acted out for Elliot and me: "The White Snake," "The Singing Bone," "The Seven Ravens," "Rapunzel," and most memorably, "The Girl without Hands." The image of the girl's stumps and the silver hands that were made for her horrified me, but those visuals were nothing compared to the images induced by the drugs I was trying to ward off. The tales worked their magic; they were so vivid that I became distracted from my fevered mental state and able to ease into the world of the fairy tales. Herbert's kind presence soothed me as well. By the time he left in the late afternoon, my mind had quieted and the demons had departed.

Although I was thoroughly exhausted and shaken, by the time my mother came home I'd returned to a normal frame of mind. But I was left with an acute awareness of how thin the veil of reality was. *Had other people experienced something like this*? I wondered. The two episodes had been so strange and frightening, I knew I couldn't talk about them with my friends or write to my father about them. Again, as with my hearing loss, I felt different from others and completely alone in this experience. There was so much I couldn't share and once again, I felt a sense of separation from my family and friends.

One thing that came out of this experience was that it instilled in me a profound respect for the power of drugs. I vowed then that I wasn't going to experiment with drugs in the future.

As my leg healed, the twins faithfully dropped by several afternoons a week to keep me company. They were a major source of connection for me, keeping me up on the gossip from school and their lives, and I lived for their visits. Finally, after five months, my cast was taken off, and I was allowed to lower my leg to the floor. I was still not supposed to put weight on it, so I spent the last two weeks of the school year transferring myself from class to class on crutches. Neila and Lynne had arranged that one of them would meet me at the door of each classroom, carry my heavy school bag filled with books, and accompany me to my next class. I treasured the intimacy of those brief conversations with them in the hallways. Just spending a few short minutes with them eased my isolation.

On the last day of school, as Neila walked me to my mother's waiting car, she burst into tears.

"What's the matter?" I asked, horrified.

"We're moving to Lafayette!" she cried. "Our parents are sending us to Acalanes High School. They think Berkeley High is too wild and that we'll get a better education at Acalanes High. But we don't want to leave Berkeley, or you. You're our best friend." Neila gulped back her sobs.

"When are you moving?" I asked. Even though I was stunned by the news, my mind had already started to jump ahead. My heart was breaking at the thought of being so far from my only two friends, and again, I would have to start another school year alone. I'd heard of Lafayette; it was fifteen miles away on the other side of the Caldecott Tunnel, but it might as well have been on the other side of the country. I didn't think either of our mothers would be willing to make the drive regularly for us to visit, and I knew I wouldn't be able to keep up with the twins through phone conversations.

"The mover's coming in a week." Neila sniffled. "Mum just told us last night, and we have to start packing."

I asked, "Can I see you this weekend, before you move?" I was numb.

"Maybe, but I'm not sure Mum will allow it. We've got so much to do."

As Neila carried my books down the stairs and opened the car door for me, I was overwhelmed by a sense of loss that had become all too familiar. Neila waved goodbye and turned to join her sister. As I watched them walk away, I envied their twinness; no matter what happened to them, they would always have each other. Slowly, I maneuvered my way into the car after laying my crutches along the back seat and hopping on my good leg onto the passenger seat in the front. I pulled the door shut.

"The twins are moving next week to Lafayette," I burst out.

"Oh, that's really too bad," my mother murmured. From her sympathetic glance as she started the car, I could tell she was sorry, but her resigned comment made the reality of the situation sink in that much more.

"I don't have any friends."

"You'll find new friends. You always do."

I didn't want to think about what it would be like to start Berkeley High without a best friend. As it turned out, I would see the twins again only four or five times over the next four years. Their mother, as I guessed would be the case, was unwilling to make the drive to Berkeley, so instead my mother drove me to their house. I loved visiting them and swimming in their pool. But to my sadness, because of the infrequency of our visits, over time our close friendship gradually faded. Once again, I'd lost a precious friendship. Once again, I was alone.

Chapter Eleven

Beginning Berkeley High wasn't as difficult as I'd feared it would be without the twins. I quickly became friends with Ann, an introverted, studious girl who was in all my classes. She was an only child to older parents, and they were very protective of her. They didn't let her go out with friends without their approval, but they liked me, for I, too, was quiet and studious.

As the twins had been, Ann was interested that I wore hearing aids, and in school she often helped me navigate some of the difficulties that my hearing disability caused. After classes she patiently updated me about the homework assignments and what our teachers had said would be covered on tests. The two of us sat together every day on a bench outside during lunch, and we often studied together on the weekends. I valued her loyalty and the world felt a lot less overwhelming with her by my side. But sometimes I wished we could branch out and join some of the other groups sitting at tables around us at lunch. I was particularly drawn to the kids from the drama club, intriguing and artsy looking in their black turtlenecks and long hair. But because of my difficulty interacting within groups, I knew I wouldn't be able to break into their gatherings.

Meanwhile my mother encouraged me to join clubs, to audition for a school play, and to try to become part of a larger group of girls. And I too wanted this for myself, for I was growing bored with my predictable life of school, homework, and piano practicing. I had a nagging sense that in some way I was missing out on some vital aspect of life.

But my mother still didn't understand how much I was limited to one-on-one interactions and making friends with loyal, quiet girls, nor did she understand how this limitation got in the way of my being able to participate in more social and exciting activities. I was torn between my mother's desires for me to build a social life and my pained awareness of my inability to tune in with my peers. I wanted to grow, but I also wanted the comfort of my safe, familiar life. I couldn't talk to my mother about this for I knew she would insist I tell people I was severely hard of hearing. I was still too ashamed to do that.

I also believed that even if I told people I couldn't understand them, it wouldn't help matters. Even if I told them about my hearing issues—which might at least make them understand why I sometimes seemed "out of it"—I knew they weren't going to consistently take care to slow down, speak one at a time, and look directly at me. I knew that this was an impossible demand of rowdy adolescent kids. I didn't want to appear to be asking for special favors by requesting a seat in the front row of the classroom, and I didn't want to interrupt a teacher's lecture repeatedly with a "What? Can you repeat that please?" Also, by now I had hidden my disability from this group of kids since middle school, and I didn't want to suddenly "come out" with the news that I was severely hard of hearing and wore hearing aids. I wasn't yet ready to advocate for myself, so I kept my peers in the dark.

I also continued to protect my mother from my pain. She had enough troubles of her own raising us as a single mother and taking care of her mother as well. I knew she wanted me to be social and outgoing, and I tried, but out of a desire to have her feel good about my life I didn't share with her most of my frustrations. So, both at home and at school, my invisible disability was making *me* invisible.

But by now I had learned the art of the bluff. At parties and in other situations, I pretended I knew what was going on by faking a smile or chuckle as others joked and laughed. This strategy allowed me to "pass" in certain situations, but I paid a price for faking it. While my inauthenticity allowed me not to draw attention to myself, ultimately those performances—and the invisibility they created—caused me even deeper loneliness.

Virtually everything other teenagers were interested in continued to be inaccessible to me. As I couldn't understand the lyrics on the radio, I had absolutely no understanding of the rock and roll music that my classmates were always talking about. Same with the television. If the conversation did turn to rock music or television programs, sometimes I pretended to know what my friends were talking about by faking a smile and then shunting aside my feelings of inauthenticity. I wondered if other kids also sometimes faked responses to fit into a group.

Movies on the big screen offered the same challenges that television shows did because I couldn't follow the dialogue, but I took great pleasure in the visual beauty of the photography that unfolded on the large screen. If the actors faced outwards towards the viewers and if there was no voice-over narration, I could lipread enough to follow some of the story. Then one day when my mother took me and Ann to the magical French movie, *Children of Paradise*, I was thrilled to discover that foreign films were subtitled. For the first time, I could understand everything that was happening onscreen. *Finally*, I was on a level playing field as everyone else in the audience. I was determined to seek out more foreign films.

Despite my social difficulties, I plunged with enthusiasm into my classes. I particularly loved English where we were working our way through Robert Graves's *The Greek Myths*, learning about the human-like adventures and misdeeds of Zeus, Hera, Apollo, Athena, and many of the other Greek gods. In class I would stare out the window gazing through the gray fog at the athletic field, imagining a misty Mt. Olympus where the gods of the ancient world directed human affairs. By happenstance I was assigned to the front row in that class, and so when Mrs. Rains asked me questions I was able to answer. I could tell she liked me, and I often lingered after class to talk with her. She recommended more books for me to read, turning me on to Charles Dickens with the suggestion I start with *Great Expectations*. Late at night my mother would come into my room to admonish me, yet again, to turn off my reading light and go to sleep, but I could tell she was secretly pleased by my reading.

I also loved freshman geometry, which I had first thing in the morning. All of us idolized our teacher, Mr. Martin, a kindly silver-haired man with warm brown eyes and black eyebrows, and I looked forward to getting out of bed early every morning to see him. At our first class he gave us each a silver compass, a protractor made of clear plastic, and a pad of graph paper. Feeling sophisticated with my new possessions, I added them to my red zippered pouch along with my pencils, pens, and eraser. I was able to follow his class well, as his talks were based on the textbook, which I'd always study the night before. He paced slowly up and down the rows of the classroom, often bending down to help us, and I could hear his explanations clearly when he corrected my problems. I enjoyed drawing arcs and circles with my new compass and calculating the angles of the various geometric shapes with my protractor. I found the predictable and ordered world of geometry soothing; I felt great satisfaction when everything added up. But more than that, in Mr. Martin's class I didn't struggle to understand what he was saying, which meant I could relax enough to enjoy learning.

During study hall and most of my spare time, I continued to passionately read the classics by English and French authors. On the bus rides home, I retreated into my books. The loud roar of the bus and the piercing, high-pitched screeches of the brakes made it impossible for me to interact with any of the rowdy kids seated around me. Ducking my head into my book, I could shut out the world and lose myself as I followed the marriage of Charles and Emma Bovary and the adventures of Dr. Manette and Charles Darnay. The characters became my friends.

In addition to the sheer pleasure of reading, I also knew it offered a great way to continue developing my language skills. My speaking vocabulary still wasn't as developed as my peers because I had trouble following complex dialogue. I felt unsophisticated and often didn't have the words to articulate what I wanted to express, which left me frustrated. But reading novels increased my vocabulary and taught me about the world—how people behaved and what they thought and felt.

One afternoon in November, my mother asked me to help clean out and tidy her clothes closet. As I rearranged her dresses, I noticed there were three new ones I hadn't seen before. Pulling them out to look more closely I noticed, shocked, that they were maternity dresses. I glanced over at my mother who was watching me closely. Suddenly I understood—she was pregnant!

"Are you . . . ?" I couldn't quite finish my question, but she blushed and nodded shyly.

I threw my arms around her. I realized then that having me discover her dresses was her way of telling me about her pregnancy. "When'll the baby be born?"

"In April," she replied.

I could hardly wait.

The following weekend John came over with boxes of his belongings and officially moved into our house. Four months later, my half-sister, Monica, was born, and as we all adored her, she pulled our little family together. When she was an infant, we put her in a baby seat on the dining room table so we could watch her gurgle and bounce up and down while we ate. Elliot and I loved to feed Monica and jostle her

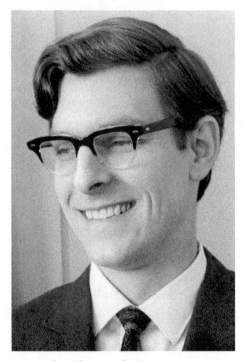

John; photo credit: Ernst Anman

about on our knees while she shrieked with delight. We could hardly wait to come home from school to babysit whenever my mother had to run out to shop for groceries and do errands. My mother stopped her work as a social worker for the next four years to stay home with Monica, and during that time she was relaxed and cheerful. Instead of the tears I witnessed during her marriage to my father, she beamed a light-heartedness I'd never seen in her before. A burden that I didn't know I had was lifted from my shoulders. With relief I thought, *I don't have to worry about her happiness and financial stresses anymore.*

One afternoon I found my mother cradling Monica in her lap, singing her a lullaby. Monica beamed and gurgled up at her.

"You know, when you were a baby I sang to you too," she said to me. "But you didn't respond at all to my singing. I didn't know then that you couldn't hear me. I just thought that's how some babies were. But then, when Elliot came along and I sang to him, he was so happy and waved his arms and babbled along with me. I just assumed he was a more social baby."

A pang pierced my heart at the image of me as a baby not hearing the sound of my mother's singing. And I wondered how many other important things I missed during my mother's early attempts to communicate with me before I received my first hearing aid. I knew she showed love through cuddling and eye gazing, but I never experienced her cooing, speaking, and singing to me. Did my inability to hear my mother's sweet, intimate sounds in a subtle way affect my early bonding with her? Had the communication problems I had with her in childhood and later been rooted in my earliest days?

For three years as my family in Berkeley grew and settled in, my father and I communicated through letters. He wrote every two weeks, sometimes asking us how we were doing at school and about our activities, but mostly he wrote of his various enterprises and obsessive projects. I wished he were more actively engaged in my life, and despite his limitations I continued to miss him with a dull ache.

Then one afternoon, quite unexpectedly, my mother told me her dear childhood friend, Maria Stolze, who lived in Munich, had written to invite me to visit her family for summer vacation. My mother had not seen Maria since she left Germany for the United States in 1947, but the two of them had kept up an active correspondence and close friendship over the years. The plan was that I would stay with Maria's family, and I'd regularly visit my father, who lived only a short bike ride away. I flung my arms around my mother in excitement. Going to Germany for the summer would be a thrilling adventure in a place I'd heard about all my life, and I'd see my father again for the first time in three and a half years.

Chapter Twelve

For the flight from San Francisco to Munich I wore a beige knit suit, a green and blue silk scarf that matched my eyes, and a navy blue French beret. I even had matching beige suede shoes with low heels, and for the first time ever, I wore stockings. In my seat I felt the smooth, sensuous glide of the nylons as I tentatively swished my calves back and forth. My mother had splurged on the outfit for the trip; I suspected she wanted me to make an impression on my father. I realized I looked older than my fourteen years when, during the fuel stop in Quebec, the middle-aged man sitting next to me offered me a cigarette from the inner pocket of his elegant suit, his lighter ready in his hand. I shyly declined.

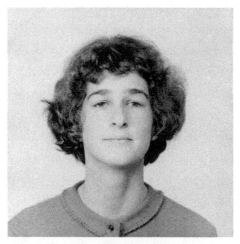

Passport photo, age fourteen

It was my first plane flight, and I pressed my nose to the window gazing at the clouds below. I was in awe of the expanse and hugeness of our world and was distracted from my small worries and concerns. After a while, the flight attendants made several announcements over the intercom system, which, between the din of the propeller and my not being able to lipread, were impossible for me to understand. I hoped they weren't telling us anything important.

I could hardly wait to see my father again, but I was also nervous. Many times over the past three years I had longed for him, missing him with a dull physical ache in my heart. I had conflicted memories; he loomed as a dark, melancholic presence in the backdrop of my life, but at the same time I could also feel his warmth and love for me. When I had last seen him, I was an eleven-year-old child with long braids and bangs and a tomboy's wiry body. Now I was much taller—a slim, awkward teenager with short curly brown hair that hid my two hearing aids. But more importantly, I wasn't sure I could share many of my thoughts and feelings about my life, and about his abruptly leaving us for Germany. Would we be able to take up where we had left off more than three years ago?

The sky turned a vibrant cobalt blue as we soared over the glittering ice fields of Greenland, and I thought about my friend, Ann, who was also traveling alone to visit friends of her family in Germany. We had spent many afternoons after school, high in the crabapple tree in my backyard, fantasizing about our upcoming trips. But I was having trouble reconciling the split feelings I had developed about Germany, the *good Germany* and the *bad Germany*. On the positive side, so much wonderful music and literature came from this country. Omama had often reminisced about the beauty of Germany, its mountainous landscape, lush forests, and elegant cities. And Germany, I knew, was where the Brothers Grimm collected their fairy tales. Many afternoons Elliot and I had sprawled out, enthralled, on the floor of my bedroom as Omama recited them, theatrically waving her arms about. She had brought from

Germany leather-bound books of esteemed German poets and play-wrights, including Goethe, Schiller, Heine, and Holderlin, and translated some of their poems for us. And in the past year I had been devouring the novels of Thomas Mann, a famous German author whose work I adored. Then there was the beauty of German music. From listening to my parents' records with my head pressed against the speakers to my own experience of playing the piano, I developed a deep love of classical music. Many of those composers were German.

Yet, as I was growing up, my parents and Omama had described the atrocities committed by the Germans during World War II. Omama and my mother had spent the war evading capture by the Nazis, but my mother's cousins, aunts, and uncle, as well as many of her classmates, perished in Theresienstadt and Auschwitz. I often wondered how this could be the same Germany that produced so much beautiful literature and music.

Sometimes, when parents of my friends asked me if we were French because of my last name, I told them that my parents were German. Upon hearing this some adults would stiffen coldly, particularly the Jewish ones. It was not that long after World War II, and there was still a lingering prejudice in America against the Germans for Germany's role in the war. I wasn't mature enough to explain that my mother was half Jewish and that my father had been active in an underground movement that fought against the Nazis. It all seemed too complicated to discuss at that time in my life.

As the plane began its descent towards the Munich airport, I took in with pleasure the lush green Bavarian countryside, the red-tiled rooftops of the houses, and the *Zwiebelkopf*—or onion shaped—domes of the churches below. My palms grew damp, and my heart beat faster at the thought of seeing my father and meeting Maria and Helmut Stolze.

Maria was my mother's best friend from childhood. It was her idea that I spend that summer in Munich with her, her husband

Helmut, and their younger daughter Regula, who at eighteen was finishing her last year of high school. I wondered why my father had never suggested that Elliot and I visit him for a summer. Did he not have the money to pay for our flights, or could he just not be bothered to extend himself to us? My mother felt I'd be happier living with the Stolzes that summer while periodically visiting my father, rather than stay with him in his apartment. As I didn't want to be alone with his heavy presence, I was fine with this arrangement.

After the plane landed in Munich, I eagerly cleared customs and hurried through the swinging doors to where my father was waiting. Older and greyer than when I last saw him, he looked shocked as he lay eyes on me. I ran towards him and he folded me into his arms, murmuring into my cheek, "My Claudia, oh my Claudia."

The Stolzes stood awkwardly to the side, looking a bit uncomfortable as they waited for my reunion with my father to leave an opening. Maria wore a blue Bavarian dirndl and apron matching her friendly blue eyes, and her blonde hair was swept up into a bun. Helmut was very tall with broad shoulders and had a cheerful, booming voice. I liked them immediately. From my mother, Maria knew of my hearing loss and spoke to me clearly in simple German. Having studied German in ninth grade, I was largely able to follow her simple greetings. But Helmut was harder to understand; he assumed my German was better than it was, and he spoke with a Bavarian accent. But he was so enthusiastic and welcoming that my heart went out to him.

After making arrangements with my father to pick me up the next evening, the Stolzes drove me to their home in the lush, leafy neighborhood of Bogenhausen near the Englisher Garten, considered one of the largest and most beautiful urban public parks in the world. Their eighteen-year-old daughter Regula met us at the front door and gave me a big hug. She told me she'd heard so much about our mothers' close friendship growing up together in Munich during the war and so she was eager to meet me. She took me up the steep staircase to her older sister's bedroom, which would be mine for the next five weeks. As I settled in for the night under a plush down comforter, I was happy. Finally, I was seeing the Germany I'd heard so much about, and I was relieved that the Stolzes were so friendly.

The next evening my father escorted me to a lavish restaurant that specialized in wild game from the nearby forests. We sat in the plush dining room lined with red velvet–paneled walls; the mounted head of an elk with grand antlers gazed dolefully down at me as we ate. Right away my father launched into a tirade about the upcoming West German federal elections to be held that fall. Having heard so many of his rants about German politics in his letters, I quickly became bored and tried to change the subject. Staring down at my remaining venison and wild rice I wondered aloud, "What does the restaurant do with all the leftover food?"

"That's an excellent question, let's ask."

When the waitress came by, my father swept his hand over our plates and then banged his knuckles so hard on the table so that the water glasses shook.

"My daughter has a very important question for you," he said, then turned towards me. "Claudia, ask the maître d' your question." I stared, red-faced, into my plate. There was no way I'd ask this question and I wasn't confident enough with my German to pose it even if I had wanted to.

As I sat in silence, my father practically yelled, "What do you do with the leftover food? Throw it out, eat it yourselves, feed it to the pigs, or give it to the poor people?"

Bowing obsequiously the waitress answered, "I don't know, but I'll get the maître d', Herr Doktor Marseille."

I scowled at my father to stop him, but when the maître d' arrived he declared, "My daughter has a very important question for you."

He turned towards me. "Claudia, ask the maître d' your question." I kicked my father under the table; I wanted this conversation to end.

"What do you do with the leftover food?" he repeated, still yelling.

The maître d', completely flustered, tried to placate my father but didn't answer the question. My father demanded, "Why can't you answer my daughter's simple question?"

People at neighboring tables were now staring openly at us and whispering amongst themselves. The maître d', tightlipped, left our table and shortly came back with two servings of *Apfelstrudel* with whipped cream. "On the house," he said coolly. I was no longer hungry, and I wanted to sink through the floor as my father lectured me on what had just happened.

"See how most people are really quite silly?" said my father. "They don't think for themselves, and few dare to speak the truth. This is how the Nazis came to power. And did you notice the strict hierarchy among the staff—how subservient the waitress was to the maître d'? They're all just like sheep!"

I could hardly wait to leave the restaurant. Here it was again, that completely familiar and generally awful divide I knew so well between my love for my father and a repulsion for his belligerent behavior. My body roiled with these conflicting emotions, and I understood more than ever why my mother had left him.

By the time I saw him again a few days later, I was feeling bold enough to ask him how, working very limited hours at his private practice as a psychoanalyst, he could have made enough money to pay off his substantial debts in the United States, move to Munich, buy a car, and rent an apartment.

"Remember *Project X?*" he said. "That's how I did it. Your clever daddy figured out a way to count cards at blackjack and slowly I made a million dollars. I was able to pay off my debts, but mostly I have been using this money to prosecute Nazi war criminals. Unfortunately, I have been unsuccessful at this. I have not made a single conviction."

I was impressed that he had made a million dollars at blackjack, or so he claimed. But despite all the money he'd made, our mother had received virtually no financial support from him in the past years, and at this point I was completely uninterested in hearing more about *Project X* or his unsuccessful campaign to prosecute war criminals. Over the years I'd had quite enough of his grandiose schemes, and here he was, admitting that despite having a substantial amount of money in his pocket, he saw fit to send us nothing, not a penny to support his children.

Over the next few weeks, the Stolzes, sometimes accompanied by Regula, drove me around Munich to see the Marienplatz, the historic city center, the late Gothic Frauenkirche, and the Old Masters paintings at the Alte Pinakothek and the Lenbachhaus. We attended classical music concerts at the Herkulesaal and made several day trips to swim in the nearby lakes of Ammersee, Tegernsee, and Schliersee in Upper Bavaria. I was enchanted by Munich's beauty, its lush surroundings, and the medieval art in its museums. But most of all I relished the loving attention I was getting from the Stolzes, very different from my interactions with my father.

One day they took me to the Baroque palace, Schloss Nymphenburg (Castle of the Nymphs), the primary summer residence of the former rulers of Bavaria, which was situated near the neighborhood in Munich where my mother grew up.

Maria told me that as a child she would take the streetcar from Munich's city center to my mother's house to play, and how in the afternoons they would wander with their bicycles in the lush park of Schloss Nymphenburg.

"Sometimes we hid in the bushes behind lovers who were making out," she said with a chuckle, "and then we would jump out and scream at them, scaring them, and then we would race off on our bicycles."

I was mesmerized when Maria explained that during the bombing of Munich my mother repeatedly climbed up on the roof of her family home and doused out the fires in the roof beams. My mother—so spunky and courageous. Maria's stories felt like gifts.

As my mother's parents had been, the Stolzes were anthroposophists, followers of the Austrian philosopher and educator Rudolf Steiner. Steiner had innovative ideas about revitalizing agriculture, education, and the Christian religion. He developed the curriculum for Waldorf schools to educate children through the arts, music, and dance, and the Stolzes' daughters, Regula and Veronika, had attended Munich's Waldorf school.

The Stolzes were different from any family I had known back in Berkeley. Regula and Veronika drew, painted, arranged flowers, played classical piano and recorder well, read poetry to each other, baked, and sewed a lot of their own clothes. This all seemed almost too good to be true, but I watched with a little sadness at how relaxed and easy the girls were with their mother, often snuggling and laughing freely with her on the couch. In the evenings, Helmut played Bach flute sonatas accompanied on the piano by Regula. Some evenings I proudly played the piano for them. And on other evenings Veronika, tall, blond, glamorous, and studying German literature at the University of Tübingen, would discuss with Helmut the poems she had to analyze for her degree. I was touched, and a bit envious, of the way Helmut was helping his daughter. So unlike my father.

One afternoon, to my delight, Maria and her daughters decided I needed an elegant party dress as part of my wardrobe. We all drove to an enormous fabric store in downtown Munich, and with their encouragement, I picked out a teal green raw silk material that matched my eyes. That evening I stood slim in my slip as Maria, holding pins in her pursed lips, expertly adjusted the paper pattern to fit me. After two more fittings, she finished the dress. It was sleeveless with a round, scooped neck and a full skirt with a belt made of the same fabric. I was delighted and touched by her act of love.

The warmth that radiated from the Stolzes affected me deeply. I lapped up their attention and I wished I could stay longer with them.

At the beginning of ninth grade, a year before my trip, my German teacher had paired the class with German pen pals. I was assigned to Ilse from Munich, and we'd been writing to each other for the past year. She wrote in German and I in English, and we agreed I'd phone her soon after my arrival in Munich to arrange a meeting.

I'd always had difficulties on the phone because I couldn't supplement with lipreading the soft and garbled sounds I heard being spoken. And when I didn't know the context of the conversation, it was even harder to figure out what was being said. Our phone at home in Berkeley had a volume adaptor on the handset and I had a switch on my hearing aid that I could press to "T-coil" mode to boost the magnetic signals from the telephone. Without a T-coil, the phone volume was simply too low for me to hear.

I stood in the Stolzes' living room and dialed Ilse's number, but when Ilse and I tried to talk, I couldn't hear her. To my dismay I realized my telecoil didn't work with the German phone system, and the Stolzes, of course, didn't have a volume adaptor on their phone. I called out to Maria and thrust the phone at her. She graciously took over and made arrangements to drive me to Ilse's house the next day. I was grateful for her help but also frustrated and embarrassed at my dependency.

The next day I met Ilse. She was tall and plain with short, frizzy light brown hair and very thick glasses. *Oh, she, too, has a disability,* I thought. *Maybe we can make a connection.* She led the way to her room where we sat on her bed to talk, but I couldn't understand her Bavarian accent and so we switched to English. But we struggled to find something to talk about, and because the encounter already felt so awkward, I didn't tell her I wore hearing aids.

Finally, Ilse's mother came into the bedroom to take me back to the Stolzes' house. She gave me a quick hug while clasping the side of my head in both of her hands and accidentally knocked out one of my hearing aids, which went flying across the wooden floor where it landed with a thud, whistling its loud feedback screech. Ilse and her mother stared at me in shock. The hearing aid was fine, but as I put it back on, I folded in on myself in mortification. Our language barrier and my disability made it impossible for us to connect and Ilse and I never contacted each other again.

I rode Regula's bicycle two or three times a week for the twenty-minute ride to my father's apartment. We took long companionable walks together in the Englisher Garten and sometimes ate at the same restaurant we'd gone to our first night together where I avoided making eye contact with the maître d'. But over games of chess back in his apartment, my father, while waiting for me to make my move, ranted on about the politics of Germany and the University of Munich, Freudian theory, Karl Marx, communism, and his failed attempts at finding patients who would be interested in taking LSD. I wanted him to pay more attention to me and once again ended up frustrated and disappointed in our interaction, much of which bored me. I relished his occasional flashes of warmth and humor, but it was no longer enough. I didn't have the father I longed for, a father who fully supported and guided me. As hard as it was to accept, I realized that he simply wasn't going to change.

Chapter Thirteen

Halfway through the summer, it was time for me to leave for a camp in the Harz Mountains near East Germany that the Stolzes and my mother had enrolled me in. They told me the Christian camp, which was focused on the arts, would give me a great opportunity to spend three weeks with German kids my age. As the train pulled through the countryside to the little town of Goslar, I was anxious about how I'd communicate, given my hearing disability and my minimal German. But I was also excited about the prospect of making new friends and taking the drawing and painting classes the camp offered. This was going to be an adventure, and I was going to embrace it. The camp was an anthroposophical camp, part of one of Rudolf Steiner's Christian Communities.

"What does that mean, Christian Community?" I had asked my mother before I left for Germany.

She explained that my grandparents were disciples of Steiner; they had attended his lectures on education and religion in Munich, and my mother had been part of the Christian Community as she was growing up. She idolized it, treasuring the lifelong friendships she made, the poetry they read, and the plays they performed.

"Omama is Jewish," I said. "Why did she have you follow a Christian path?"

"Omama and her family didn't observe any Jewish practices," she explained. "They had assimilated into German society, so for her it felt natural to follow anthroposophy and participate in the Christian Community."

During World War II, my mother explained, the Nazis banned the Christian Communities and Waldorf schools as they didn't adhere to Nazi ideology and were associated with people like freemasons, Jews, and pacifists who were a threat to their goals. But since the end of the war, the Christian Community and the Waldorf schools had made a comeback.

"I know you'll just love the camp because of all the arts and because Maria's daughters loved it too," my mother had promised.

But things were off to a bad start; when I stepped off the train in the late afternoon in the little village of Goslar, it was pouring rain. Through the thick gray clouds, I couldn't see the low range of the Harz mountains with their rolling foothills of forests and green fields. A camp counselor met a group of us at the station and drove us the short distance by van to the camp, which consisted of a grand former hunting lodge built of brown timber, now converted into several dormitories.

I was assigned to a large room with seven other girls from a Waldorf school in Munich who had arrived earlier that day and had already claimed their bunk beds. As soon as I entered the room, I could tell from their intimate conversations that the girls already knew each other and were good friends. I tried to insert myself into their conversations, but I couldn't understand their answers. After they realized I couldn't converse easily with them, they lost interest in me and I watched in misery as they left the room and strolled arm-in-arm through the building. There was no natural opening for me to tell them I was hard of hearing, particularly as I had studied German only for one year. The first night it was all I could do to hold back my tears as the girls happily chattered in the dark. I wanted to run for the next train back to the Stolzes.

The following morning, we had to sign up for different activities. I couldn't understand the different options that the director read rapidly in German amidst the shouting of the kids surrounding him. I understood only that one option was a mime group, which I knew would be easier for me than some of the others as it would involve little speaking, but by the time I figured out where to sign up, the mime class was full. *Maybe I can join the recorder group,* I thought; I played the recorder well and, again, the focus would be on the music and not on having to talk or strain to listen to speech. But that class also was full, along with the drawing and painting classes. My heart sank as I was assigned to the last class still open, the stained-glass class. I knew nothing about stained-glass, and the idea of assembling bits of glass into a design didn't appeal to me at all. After our assignments, it was time for lunch.

The dining room, which had a high wood beam ceiling and windows that overlooked a wet, misty meadow and muddy soccer field, was cheerfully decorated with floral curtains and bouquets of wildflowers on the tables. But the roar of kids talking and shouting all at once in German was excruciatingly garbled, and my attempts to follow the many conversations whooshing around me were hopeless. My mouth went dry, and I couldn't eat.

Nighttime was the worst. In the darkness I couldn't make out what the girls were whispering and giggling in their bunk beds. Probably about boys, I guessed. I desperately wanted to join the conversations but that being impossible, I placed my open book facedown over my hearing aids on the nightstand to hide them and pretended to be asleep. With my eyes closed tight, I tried to conjure happy memories to comfort myself. I thought about the Stolzes, who had included me in their family circle and made me feel I mattered. I tapped into memories of past Christmases with our beautiful tree decorated with red candles and gold tinsel, when Elliot and I still lived with my parents and grandmother in Berkeley.

To my great surprise, the mornings spent creating stained-glass-work turned out to be an oasis of silence, beauty, and color—a balm to my wrenched heart. We worked quietly, soldering together fragments of colored glass onto a clear glass base. I created a bright underwater world of goldfish swimming in different shades of blue and aqua water in a background of seaweed and palm fronds. Eventually I looked around to see what the other kids were working on. I was shocked to see that they were each working on an image of Mary, Mother of Jesus, standing clad in a red dress with a blue robe, replete with a halo around her head. Clearly, I hadn't understood the instructions that first day, but nobody had said anything. My cheeks reddened with embarrassment, but I continued working on my cheerful fish.

Apart from the morning respite of the class, the days slogged on interminably. It continued to rain, the gunmetal gray skies adding to my depression as I drifted like a ghost through the days. It reminded me of how I'd felt during my first lonely weeks of eighth grade two years earlier. No one approached me, and I didn't know how to break into any of the cliques that formed around me. The staff had no idea I was hard of hearing, and my counselor was too distracted to notice much of anything as she was involved in a summer romance with one of the counselors from the boy's camp. Again, I thought with despair, I was in over my head; my mother hadn't notified the camp of my hearing disability, and I was too embarrassed to do so myself. And in addition to my marginal German, telling them probably wouldn't make any difference in my ability to participate.

The camp director promised us mushroom hunting, hiking, and soccer as soon as the weather cleared, but as the days passed the downpour pounding on the roof showed no sign of abating. The other kids seemed happy enough singing songs and putting on skits, but I couldn't sing along with them as I couldn't make out the lyrics because of the varying pitches of the vowels, which distorted the words. And worse still, the songs were in German. Because I was so quiet, I was afraid the others thought I was slow. This frustrated me because I knew that I was actually not particularly shy and certainly not slow.

I just didn't know how to speak up about my limitations. As a result, they barely saw me, and I just passed by quietly in the fringes.

After a few days, the kids started rehearsing a play to be performed for Parents' Visiting Day at the end of camp. My father had assured me before I left for camp that he would visit me, and I wrote to him reminding him of his promise and asked him to come for the performance. I wanted a role in the play, but all the parts were assigned already. One afternoon the theater director spotted me standing off to the side and gave me the role of the silent maid who came and went, bringing food and drinks to the other characters in the play. Happy to be included as part of the production, I didn't mind my role and was pleased with my costume of a peasant dress with apron and frilly cap. I'd absolutely no idea what the play was about or even what it was called, but I didn't want to tell anyone how clueless I was.

Along with the stained-glass workshop, reading was my lifeline. While other kids were singing together or rehearsing their skits, I sequestered myself in a corner or retreated to my bunk bed and read *The Magic Mountain* by Thomas Mann, about a young man who spends seven years in the rarified world of a tuberculosis sanatorium high in the Swiss Alps. I didn't understand it all back then, didn't realize that through his characters, Mann was representing a microcosm of pre-World War I Europe, nor did I totally understand his references and meditations on the philosophy of time, German thought, and Goethe and his writings, but I understood enough to be fascinated. I savored the escape to the world Thomas Mann created high in the mountains. In Mann I found a friend, and I really needed one.

As comforting as reading was, it made me feel guilty; when I withdrew to read, I could hear my mother's voice, "Join the other kids and have fun!" She had high hopes that the camp would be a good experience. She wanted me to be someone I couldn't be—cheerful and more social. I tried to be that for her, to be as normal as possible. But in recent years I'd begun to feel less and less normal. As usual, despite my unhappiness at camp, in my letters I didn't write to my mother what I was going through. I didn't lie; I simply didn't tell her how difficult the camp experience was. I was always conscious of the fact that no matter what hardships I experienced, it was nothing compared to her suffering in Nazi Germany. I held onto that perspective for years, and it made me go through periods in my childhood and young adulthood ashamed of my depression and protective of my mother's feelings. I wondered how often children, out of loyalty, protected their parents from their pain.

As the days at camp dragged on, I couldn't snap out of my unhappiness. A sodden gray misery had seeped into my very pores, and I continued to feel like a ghost leaving no trace on Earth. I wondered whether hearing disabled people were more prone to anxiety and depression because of the isolation that results from deafness.

Years later, I did some research and came across a number of papers, including a 2014 study by the National Institute for Deafness and other Communication Disorders, which found a strong link between hearing loss and depression. Difficulty in communicating with others often results in loneliness, social isolation, and depression. Because we're an interdependent and social species, being cut off from our fellow humans can be painful; at its most extreme, it can threaten our survival. While my survival was not literally at stake, I felt cast from the circle of human contact, friendship, and love.

When it was time to start a second stained-glass project, we were told to work on a subject of our choosing, and I decided to create a Mother Mary figure as everyone else had done. At first I felt a little strange working on a Mary as I'd had virtually no religious education, but as I worked, inserting blue glass for her dress, I was comforted. She seemed to radiate back to me love and compassion that I so needed. Choosing and inserting just the right shiny, reflective pieces of glass into my piece in the silence of the room felt healing. Those mornings offered a magnificent surprise. Apart from brief escapes into reading, creating a magical world out of jewel-colored glass while the rain streamed down the windowpanes was the only time during the interminable days and nights that I wasn't consumed by a debilitating anxiety and misery in my belly.

On Parent's Visiting Day, the building buzzed with excitement as parents arrived from all around Germany and hugged and kissed their campers. I hadn't received a letter back from my father, but I hoped he would arrive in time to watch the performance of our play that afternoon. *He's never seen me on stage before. He will be amused to see me in my maroon dress,* I thought. Finally, the play began, the makeshift red blanket curtain swung open, and I walked out from the wings carrying a platter of wine glasses to a table set in the middle of the stage. I stood quietly for several minutes as the others spoke and gesticulated, searching around the room among the faces in the audience for that of my father. Gradually, when with a sinking heart I realized he wasn't among the other parents, I fought to keep back my tears. When I returned to my room after the play, there was a letter from him waiting on my bed. He explained that he would very much have liked to have seen me but that he was too busy writing an "important article on Lorenz's theory of aggression" and couldn't take the time to come and visit. I tore up the letter and threw the pieces in the wastebasket.

That night I was particularly miserable. My tongue wandered over the painful canker sores that had formed the past few days on my gums and inside my cheeks. I wondered if they were from my dry mouth and not being able to eat much the past three weeks. I tried to console myself by visualizing good times with my father. I missed him in a dark and heavy-hearted way, but as with my mother, I couldn't write to him the extent of my misery; I didn't want him to be disappointed in me and at my inability to stay cheerful in a challenging situation. I realized he was completely preoccupied with his own projects and was only superficially interested in how I was adjusting socially or academically. I knew he couldn't make my problems go away, but I wished he at least would have visited and supported me, as the other parents did.

When at last I returned to Munich and Maria met me at the station, I could hardly hold back my tears of relief and gratitude at her warm, enveloping hug. She exclaimed with sympathy when I showed her my mouth full of sores and she remarked with concern that I'd lost weight. She wanted to hear about the camp, but I didn't tell Maria the truth of my experience. Along with my mother it had been her idea that I attend the camp, and she'd told me how much I'd enjoy it. I didn't want her to feel badly by telling her how helpless and miserable I had been. But when we drove up to the house, I was thrilled to see that Regula had draped the front door with a streamer that read "*Willkommen!*" and had decorated the house and my room with wildflowers she had collected. Helmut, Maria, and Regula all hugged me as they guided me into the house, and with a profound relief I felt the deep anxiety of the past three weeks leave my body as I was enfolded into their circle of love.

That evening I presented Maria with my stained-glass piece of Mary, wrapped in pink tissue paper and a red satin ribbon. I was excited for her to open it, and as she undid the wrapping and saw Mary glowing at her, she gasped and hugged me. At dinner I looked around at the family seated at the table around me and almost cried as they all tenderly smiled at me. Maria had made a special dinner of apricot-stuffed dumplings with a cinnamon butter sauce. I had three helpings.

"Were they Nazis during the war?" I asked. My father and I were driving to Schloss Elmau, a resort hotel high in the Bavarian Alps to spend the final two weeks of my summer together before I returned home to Berkeley, and I was full of curiosity about the owners of the resort.

"Well, probably back then some of the owner's family and guests were Nazi sympathizers, but nobody speaks of that now," he said. I was curious if I might spot some ex-Nazis at the resort and if I could tell just by looking at them.

My father had always been a horrible driver. On the drive to Schloss Elmau, he pressed his foot down on the accelerator of his little VW bug until we were speeding at 115 kilometers per hour on a two-lane road. He leaned over the steering wheel to peer over the top of the windshield to recite the names of the Alpine mountains we were approaching, and he repeatedly veered into the opposite lane, then swerved at the last instance back into his lane, nearly missing approaching cars. It seemed to be a game for him, but I was terrified and shaken.

"Please slow down," I said.

"Your daddy's an excellent driver, you'll see, I won't hit any cars."

At last, we arrived at the small castle set back in a lush green meadow. As we climbed out of the car, my father pointed and said, "Those are the snowcapped peaks I climbed when I was a teenager." I was relieved to arrive alive, enchanted by the fairytale surroundings.

The next morning as we rambled through the dark forest near the castle, he rattled on about German politics. Again, I was disappointed that he didn't ask something about me, about school, about my experience at camp, or about Elliot. The afternoons were better; we had tea with *Pflaumkuchen mit Schlagzahne* (plum cake with whipped cream) on the wide terrace overlooking the green meadow while we played dominoes and chess. I took a photograph of him on a black wrought-iron bench, his arm resting along the back, the wind blowing his wavy black hair speckled with gray, his blue eyes smiling wryly back at me. For the dance evenings in the ballroom where a pianist played old-fashioned waltzes and fox trots, I slipped on the sleeveless turquoise silk dress that Maria had sewed for me in preparation for these dances. My father danced stiffly, bowing formally and kissing my hand at the end of each dance, as was the custom. Several times, a young man would ask me to dance and we'd twirl enthusiastically around the room. I was always relieved when my partner chose not to speak as we danced, for I knew I wouldn't be able to follow what he said. But, confident in my new dress, I felt seen. The invisibility I'd experienced at camp had disappeared.

My father and I spent the next two weeks taking walks, playing tennis on the red clay courts, and playing bocce ball. I loved playing those games with him; it was my father at his best. He was encouraging and yelled "Hurrah!" whenever I made a particularly good shot or hit one of his bocce balls. When we played a game that required concentration like dominoes or chess, I had his undivided attention. In the evenings, we listened to chamber music in the concert hall where there was a decades-long rule against clapping in order to enjoy the aftermath of the music in silence.

But once, after a superb performance by Wilhelm Kempf of Beethoven's last three ethereal piano sonatas, my father insisted on jumping up and yelling "Bravo, Bravo!" into the hushed hall. Everyone turned to glare at us while I, mortified, shrank into myself. Afterwards, over a game of chess, I asked him, "Why can't you just conform to a simple social convention to keep silent?"

"We shouldn't blindly follow rules that don't make sense," he said.

"These are not the Nazis, and I think it makes sense to sit in silence for a moment."

"Acknowledging a superb performance by clapping makes more sense. You'll see as you get older that most people are asleep, they are sheep and won't think for themselves. Speaking up for your beliefs against silly rules is important, and if you want to change things you have to start somewhere," he said.

My father's protests against the Nazis before World War II may have been admirable at that time, but as I had witnessed growing up, he was unwilling to adjust to the norms of post-war society, like making mortgage payments, paying taxes, and earning a living to support his family. I knew it was futile to argue. Again, I found it difficult to reconcile my divided heart. I was pulled between my love for him but also my aversion to his dark moods, inflexibility, and self-absorption.

When the summer drew to a close and it was almost time for me to return to Berkeley, I spent a last few delightful days with the Stolzes, swimming in a nearby alpine lake. My father picked me up when it was time to leave for the airport and stood by awkwardly as the Stolzes enveloped me in tight hugs. I had a hard time pulling away from them; I knew I would miss the warmth of their family and their easy expressions of love and attention. *So unlike my father*, I thought. At the airport I noticed my father looked tired and drawn. He didn't say a word as we checked my suitcase and watched it glide down the chute. I wanted to get away from him, to shake his heavy presence from me, but at the same time I loved him. I thought with misery, *I have no idea when my next visit will be.*

As he hugged me goodbye he broke into choked sobs. "I don't know when I'll see you again. Goodbye, my dear Claudia," he gasped, pressing me hard to him, tears on his cheeks.

My body stiffened as he hugged me, and I turned my face away from his cheek. I was shocked at the fury that coursed through my body at witnessing his grief. I had a hard time containing my mixed emotions, grief at having to bear the burden of his sorrow as well as my own. And anger that he seemed so unwilling to change. He didn't suggest coming to visit Elliot and me or invite us for Christmas or next summer's vacation. The few weeks I saw him that summer were as much as he could or would extend himself.

I pulled away from him and reached down to grab my carry-on satchel. Then I glanced up to take a final look. For the first time I saw him as an old man, defeated in his dark suit, with tears coursing down his sunken cheeks, dark circles under his eyes. I walked up the steps to the plane and didn't look back. But I knew he was standing there, waving at me with his white handkerchief.

Chapter Fourteen

I entered tenth grade at Berkeley High School happy to see Ann again. We were eager to reconnect and compare notes about our summers. She'd had a wonderful time with her friend in Frankfurt, so I felt I couldn't share my disastrous camp experience. I wished there was someone I could tell how awful it had been, but I felt there was nobody I could talk to about it. Instead, I told Ann all about the wonderful time I'd spent with the Stolzes in Munich and with my father at Schloss Elmau. As usual, I kept the darkest aspect of my life to myself.

I was happy to see my family again, particularly Monica, who at five months was a toothless bundle of joy. I treasured time spent bouncing her on my lap, throwing her high in the air, amidst her shrieks of laughter, and then rocking her to sleep over my shoulder. But soon my life was back in its familiar routine of school, homework, reading, piano practicing, and an occasional rendezvous with a friend on the weekend. I continued to love my piano lessons and practicing, but it was a solitary activity, and I yearned for more people in my life, more excitement, more something.

For the fall semester in PE, we were required to choose a sport; I chose tennis. My parents, tennis enthusiasts, had arranged for lessons for me and Elliot as young children, so I was already reasonably good and loved the sport. Several afternoons a week after school I changed into my white tennis shorts and ran down the hill with my racket and balls to practice at the Berkeley Rose Garden's public courts just a few blocks from our house. Rose bushes surrounded the court, and the air was redolent with sweet and spicy perfumes. I felt the satisfying pop of the ball against my racket as I practiced my stroke against the backboard, and as the weeks went by, my backhand became smoother and more consistent.

After a few weeks I noticed a tall, balding middle-aged man with watery blue eyes expertly hitting balls next to me against the backboard. I noticed his eyes focused on me and on my legs, which made me uncomfortable. One afternoon he tried to talk to me while we were both hitting balls, but I couldn't understand him without stopping my play and looking directly at him. But he was persistent, and one afternoon when we both stopped to pick up balls, he asked if I wanted to rally with him on one of the courts. I nodded, and we walked onto a court and started to play. He was an expert player and directed his balls right to me. Soon I relaxed and enjoyed the ease of playing with someone so much better than I.

When the sky began to darken, I told him I needed to get home.

"Can we play again on Friday afternoon?" he asked.

I wondered what a middle-aged man was doing playing tennis with a fourteen-year-old girl in the middle of a workweek, but I liked hitting balls with him; I was making progress. I just wished his eyelids weren't so red, his eyes such a pale, icy blue. Still, I pushed my reservations aside.

"Okay, I can come after school on Friday."

He smiled. "My name's David."

For several weeks, on Wednesday and Friday afternoons we rallied together at the Rose Garden courts. Often David would say something to me that I couldn't hear from the other side of the court, so I either I didn't respond to his comments or I just nodded. As was my way, I was too embarrassed to tell him I was hard of hearing. I hoped he didn't think I was slow.

One afternoon before we started playing, he took the balls from my hand and laid them on the ground.

"Let me show you how to improve the form of your backhand. You're not holding your racket quite right."

He surprised me by standing behind me and wrapping his arms around me. He then rotated my grip slightly counterclockwise on the racket. Several times he guided my arm, moving it through the air, his hand held firmly over mine in the correct position. He rested his chin on the top of my head. *What is he doing?* I wondered. Then suddenly from behind, he pressed me hard to him and reached around and tried to kiss my mouth. I began to panic. I turned my head away to the side, so he was only able to reach the side of my cheek. I pulled away from him and walked back out onto the court to play. After we were done rallying and it was my usual time to leave, he handed me my balls, his hand lingering on mine.

"You must be thirsty. Shall we go and get a milkshake?"

I knew there was no place nearby to get a milkshake and I would have to get in his car.

"No thanks, I don't want a milkshake." I looked at him, but his intense blue eyes piercing into me made me turn away.

"Of course you want a milkshake. What pretty young woman doesn't want a milkshake after playing tennis? What's your favorite flavor?" He stood in front of the chain- linked gate, blocking my only way off the court.

"I don't know you, and I don't want to get in your car."

"What, you don't trust me?"

His lips strained into a thin smile, and his eyes hardened. I wanted to get home. I glanced around the court, and my eyes landed on a second exit on the opposite side.

"I just don't want to get in your car," I repeated. "I have to get home now."

I tried to keep my voice steady. I looked around at the other courts but there was no one else around. The relative safety of the busy street of Euclid Avenue was far away.

"I thought you liked me. Can't I just treat you to an ice cream? Don't you trust me?" he whined.

I placed my balls into my tennis bag, slung my racket in its case over my shoulder, and turned away to get out of there. He grabbed my upper arm, his grip firm and menacing.

"I only want us to be friends," he said.

I yanked his arm off and whirled away from him. "I don't want to be friends. I have to get home."

"Then let me walk you home."

I knew better than to let him find out where I lived, so suddenly, I sprinted off the court. He yelled something after me as I ran through the tunnel connecting the Rose Garden to the Codornices playground and then into a grove of oak trees up a small rise. I waited awhile behind the trees, then, when I felt confident he wasn't following me, I ran the few blocks back to my house. *It was my fault,* I thought. *I should have known better. I brought this upon myself by agreeing to play tennis with him.* I also thought that if I'd heard him more clearly, I might have understood his intentions earlier on.

I didn't tell my family what had happened. I simply told my mother I would stop playing tennis after school for now as I had a lot of homework. For the next six months I went to the courts only on the weekends when Elliot played tennis with me. To my relief I never saw David again. I realized I'd escaped what could have been a dangerous situation and felt proud that I'd gotten away from him and hadn't led him to my home. I knew I was living in a world that was dangerous for a teenaged girl, particularly a hearing disabled one. I vowed to keep my eyes wide open.

For spring semester, I had to take swimming lessons for PE. On the first day of class I realized I'd have to get naked in front of the other girls in the locker room as we changed into our swimsuits. I noticed that many of them were changing out of lacy bras into sexy bikinis, which made me feel gawky and shy in my ill-fitting dark green one-piece suit. Mortified, not wanting anyone to see my body, I draped the small white gym towel around my shoulders as best as I could while changing into my bathing suit. I was self-conscious about how my slim body compared to many of the other girls' voluptuous curves. It wasn't until after high school when I had my first lover that I realized that men appreciated my body and that I had nothing to be self-conscious about.

But even worse, because I was still hiding my hearing aids from the world, I had to surreptitiously take them off and tuck them in my locker wrapped safely in my blouse. Now I was completely deaf. I couldn't hear the giggles and gossip that went on in the locker room or anyone address me. I was completely isolated in my own world. As fast as I could, I slinked across the locker room and out onto the pool deck.

At the pool, ahead of the other girls, I was hit with the strong smell of chlorine and the steam rising off the surface as I glided into the water and rolled over onto my back. Staring up at the industrial pipes snaking across the ceiling, I backstroked along the length of the pool. Once the class started, I carefully watched the teacher and the other kids, copying whatever they did. Mostly we swam laps. I was a strong swimmer and was pleased to be picked early for a team whenever we had relay races. I could race without anyone noticing I couldn't hear. At the end of the period, I climbed out of the pool as fast as I could, skipped the shower, and changed into my clothes before the other girls got back into the locker room. I could hardly wait to get out of that building and escape to my English class where we were reading Thomas Hardy's *Return of the Native.*

Ann told me that the class was grumbling at the slow plotting and long descriptions of the wild Wessex moors, but I couldn't get enough of the novel's story of doomed love, passion, and alienation and its melancholic atmosphere of loss and longing. Reading about the extreme troubles of others, of Eustacia's devastating marriage and then her tragic drowning, made my issues of trying to fit in seem pretty manageable. But I didn't just want to read about what happened to other people; I was biding my time, waiting for my life to change.

Ann was friends with Deborah, a pretty, confident blonde senior who, in the spring semester, told us about a school club she had just joined to learn to model clothes. It was led by Miss Berryman, a secretary at the school, and she taught proper posture, graceful walking, and makeup application. I wasn't much interested in makeup or learning proper deportment, but when Deborah asked whether Ann and I wanted to join the club and participate in the fashion show coming up in a month, we jumped on it. Modeling clothes sounded like fun. Miss Berryman phoned around to various boutiques and clothing stores and explained what the club wanted; in exchange for lending us clothes for the show, the store's name would be printed on the show's program. A number of shops agreed to participate, and appointments were scheduled for us to try on clothes after school in the following weeks.

Ann and I were assigned to visit Kaldor's Knit Shop, a store for mature women on Shattuck Avenue. Looking around the store, with its many racks of suits for older women, I was worried whether Mrs. Kaldor sold anything suitable for teenage girls, but I was excited when she rolled out a rack with some fun silky, slinky dresses for us to try on.

As we pulled different outfits on over our heads, Mrs. Kaldor fussed over us, clucking in her thick accent, "Oh, it fits you like a dreeeam, my dear," and Ann and I spent several hours in the dressing rooms whirling around for each other. I particularly loved a form-fitting raspberry-colored flapper dress that made me look quite grown-up. Mrs. Kaldor brought out a long string of fake pearls to wear with it and suggested I find a cigarette holder to complete the look. I planned to wear my mother's high-heeled silver shoes to go with the dress. I was thrilled. I felt sophisticated, a new feeling for me, I and could hardly wait for the fashion show.

At the club's next meeting we modeled our borrowed clothes for each other, and Miss Berryman showed us how to do a catwalk strut with long strides and a slight sway of our hips from side to side. The other girls discussed the music they wanted to accompany our show. I couldn't catch the names of the songs or singers they selected, and not being able to understand the words to popular music, I wouldn't have known the songs anyway. I only understood the title chosen to be the theme song: "Wild Thing." During the afternoon of our practice run-through in the high school auditorium, I was able to drop my reserved, awkward persona. I was confident I would feel the rhythm of the music even if I didn't understand the words. Strutting in my sparkly flapper dress, I twirled my long necklace and sashayed to the beat of "Wild Thing" as the other girls whooped, smiled, and clapped. The experience made me flush with feelings of belonging and acceptance.

We had our theme song, but we still needed a name for the show. As the others bandied about different possibilities, I quipped, "How 'bout *Threads for Mod Bods*?" Everyone loved it, and I was thrilled to see the programs when they arrived from the printer with my show name in bold letters on the top. A week later, when it was time for our performance, we girls excitedly lined up in the wings, peeking out as the audience filled up with our classmates, friends, and families in the large high school auditorium. The hall was packed. The stereo boomed our theme song and the audience clapped enthusiastically as we sashayed single file across the stage to the music. Backstage we helped each other through several outfit changes, all of us buzzing with energy. The excitement in the auditorium grew, the audience whooping and cheering us on. Miss Berryman, cheeks flushed, hugged each of us as we strutted off the stage. I was elated and only sorry it was over so soon. As she drove me home my mother said little about the show; this not being part of her European heritage, I suspected she found it a bit trashy. But I didn't care; I'd been part of a thrilling show. I'd been accepted into a group.

Buoyed by the success of the fashion show, I decided to join another school club, the American Friends Service (AFS) Club, a Quaker organization dedicated to promoting peace and social justice. The club was focused on making students from other countries feel welcome as they attended Berkeley High School and on developing projects to promote world peace. I thought this would be a chance for me to get to know students from abroad. I thought that kids from other parts of the world might understand what it meant not to fit in. Maybe I would make some new friends. And promoting world peace sounded like a good idea. I thought my father would approve. I still wanted to make him proud.

At our first meeting, twenty of us, half local students and half from foreign countries, sat around the circular table in one of the classrooms. A teacher, Mrs. Bendix, told us to introduce ourselves and then said that next week we should be ready to vote for a president, secretary, and treasurer. After that, she would no longer attend the meetings, but we could phone her if we wanted her advice. She wanted the club to be self-organizing and encouraged us to come up with ideas for projects we might want to take on. I was sorry that Mrs. Bendix wasn't going to be involved, for I wasn't confident that we, mostly sophomores, could run the club on our own.

At the next meeting, students suggested names of students for the various offices we were to vote on. To my surprise, Lakshmi, a friendly Indian girl I had talked with at the previous meeting, nominated me for president. No other names were proposed, and before I knew what was happening, I was elected president of the AFS Club. I felt a warm glow as I realized that people liked me enough to vote for me, but I definitely didn't want to be president. I had absolutely no idea what I'd be expected to do. Mrs. Bendix then told us we should brainstorm ideas for projects and decide which ones we wanted to take on. "I look forward to hearing your plans, and I wish you luck," she said, and with that she left the room.

I sat at the table, frozen. I mumbled, "What do we want to do?" but I couldn't follow the different conversations buzzing around the room. Some of the kids looked to me for direction, but as I hadn't a clue how to proceed, I tried to avoid making eye contact with anyone. After a few minutes, Martha, who was sitting next to me, poked me in the arm and said, "Go on, why don't you go to the blackboard and write down our ideas?" This, I knew, would be a disaster. To write on the board, I'd have my back to the group so I wouldn't be able to hear anybody's ideas. I turned to Martha and said, "Why don't *you* go up and jot down the ideas?" She looked surprised but pleased and she strode confidently to the front of the room. The rest of the meeting went by with lively discussions circulating all around me, and my face burned as I sat silent, completely lost. Eventually, everyone ignored me as they looked to Martha who was busily writing at the blackboard.

When at last the meeting finally ended, Martha passed around a sheet of paper for everyone to write down their phone numbers. Handing me the sheet she said, "I couldn't write down all the ideas. Why don't you call everyone and get their input so we can vote on them next week. You should probably call Mrs. Bendix too, to see what she thinks."

I knew that I wouldn't be able to make those phone calls. The T-coil on my hearing aids allowed me to have only very rudimentary phone conversations with Ann about what time we would get together or what the homework assignment was. I wouldn't be able to have substantive conversations with students I didn't know. I wanted to ask Martha if she would be president in my stead, but I was too humiliated to explain my predicament. I grabbed the sheet of paper from her and bolted from the room. My mother picked me up from school that afternoon. "How'd it go?" she asked with an expectant smile as I quickly slid into the seat next to her. I didn't want to disappoint her, but for once, out of desperation, I unburdened myself.

"I can't do it! I couldn't hear the other kids, and I couldn't write notes or participate in the discussion. And I can't make the phone calls to the other kids. I made a complete fool of myself."

She nodded sympathetically but didn't say anything. I thought there wasn't really anything she could do to help, but I desperately wished there was. I didn't make the phone calls and never returned to the club. I knew I was paying a great price in not telling others about my disability. My silence was hurting the quality of my relationships and my life. But I also knew that telling others—while it would help them understand why I wasn't able to fully participate—wouldn't actually make it any easier for me to function in a group. From experience I knew that expecting kids to remember to talk one at a time and look at me while speaking was unrealistic. But I also knew that if I told them what I was dealing with, at least they'd be less likely to think me dim-witted or disabled, and that made me determined to gather the courage, soon, to tell people the truth I'd been hiding much of my life.

Chapter Fifteen

One sunny afternoon that spring my mother motioned for me to sit with her at the round glass table on the front patio where a plate of blueberry Danish muffins and a pot of black tea awaited us. She smiled as she poured me a cup. Pink and yellow roses were blossoming in the flowerbeds surrounding the small lawn, and, although I couldn't hear them, I saw birds flitting about with wisps of grass in their beaks.

With a serious look in her eyes, she said, "I want to tell you more about my life growing up half Jewish in Nazi Germany." I sat up straight. She had occasionally shared fragments of stories about her life in Germany, and I was fascinated by these accounts, but she upset me when she once said, "You've nothing to complain about. You weren't in Germany during the war." I took a bite of my Danish as my mother took a sip of tea. Then she plunged right in.

"Early in 1945, Omama learned that finally the SS were planning to deport her to the Theresienstadt concentration camp. Although we were Jewish, Omama and I had survived in Munich to that point with luck and a few good Germans who helped us. But now, just at the end of the war, we couldn't be sure of anything, and our luck seemed to be running out."

My mother went on. With the increased Allied bombings of German cities during the winter of 1944–45, it was clear that the war was almost over. The Allies had landed on the beaches of Normandy the previous June of 1944, and were now, at long last, marching into Germany. But they had not yet liberated Germany, and the Nazis, even in early 1945, were still intent on killing as many remaining Jews as possible. My mother had my full attention.

"What happened to you and Omama and her family?" I asked. For all the years I'd lived with my grandmother, I'd known she was shrouded in a layer of grief for her family, but nobody had ever fully explained why.

"Well, I guess I should start at the beginning," my mother answered.

Omama was born in Prague in 1884 and was the eldest daughter of a nonobservant Jewish banker. She wanted to be an actress, and this horrified her respectable bourgeois parents, but at age eighteen Omama ran away with a theater director who set her up in his theater in Munich. She became an actress, well-known throughout Germany, and eventually she reconciled with her family back in Prague.

I already knew Omama had been famous because I had often lain on the floor of her bedroom going through her box of publicity photographs and postcards that showed her in costume as she portrayed various roles. My favorite one was of her as Ophelia, dead, lying with her hands crossed over her chest, her eyes shut and her long brown hair strewn alongside her body.

"Your grandfather, Ludwig Zeise, was one of her admirers, and, laden with armfuls of flowers, he wooed her with proposals of marriage during his frequent visits backstage." My mother smiled.

Ludwig was twelve years younger than Omama. I was intrigued by this, as my mother had married John, also twelve years her junior. Ludwig had earned an Iron Cross for bravery during WWI when he was only a seventeen-year-old lieutenant. Because of the Cross, the Nazis considered him a hero, which would later provide a considerable level of protection to his Jewish wife, Omama, and my mother. But back in 1922, Ludwig was still a student working on an obscure PhD on the concept of "Time and the German Soul." I had no idea what this PhD could be about, and I wondered how someone could possibly get a job based on such an abstract subject. Some members

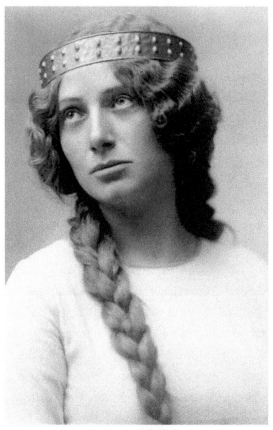

Omama as Ophelia

of Ludwig's family became Nazi sympathizers, but he defied his family by opposing the territorial and anti-Semitic policies of the Nazis. At first his parents were quite unhappy about his marriage to an older Jewish actress, but they gradually came to tolerate Omama. Ludwig eventually finished his PhD and landed a job as a psychologist testing officer candidates for the German army. Their only child, my mother, was born in 1923.

Ludwig was a socialist, but he had married a banker's daughter. This difference in their social backgrounds was a greater source of disagreement between them than Omama's being Jewish. In Prague, Omama had grown up enjoying the comforts and conveniences of having a governess, maid, and cook, but Ludwig would allow for only one maid, Kaethe, whom my mother adored.

My mother went on to say that Omama was often histrionic. During her fights with Ludwig, everyone could hear her shrieks throughout the house, and Ludwig responded to her tantrums by withdrawing, silent, to his study. *Sort of like my father,* I thought.

Often after their fights, Ludwig would leave the house and take the train to visit his parents in Berlin, but he always returned to Omama and my mother. Over the years they considered divorcing, but Ludwig didn't want this; with the rise of fascism it would've been too dangerous for him to divorce Omama, as it would have left her and my mother without the protection of a well-regarded German husband and father.

Ludwig became an anthroposophist, and my mother was enrolled in the local chapter of Steiner's Christian Community. "My youth group was wonderful. We did lots of fun activities including singing in a lovely choral group, putting on plays, and hiking in the forests of Bavaria," my mother said wistfully. "I feel sad for you that you haven't been able to make a group of friends like that at Berkeley High."

Her commentary on my social life stung. I tried to be more connected and social, but my mother didn't understand how difficult and painful it was for me to continually fail at my attempts to have a dynamic and more social high school experience with a close circle of friends. Her comparison of her social life to mine hurt, but I didn't say anything. Withholding painful truths about my life had become a habit. But ultimately this lack of authenticity did us both a disservice. I was hiding an important part of myself from my own mother.

My grandparents would have liked to have enrolled my mother at a Waldorf school, but in the early 1930s the Nazis banned the schools for being too independent of their ideology. So, in 1930, at age seven, my mother started school at a local Catholic convent where she was taught by nuns. No one at the school knew that she was half Jewish; her parents didn't reveal this to the authorities, and my mother was very firmly told not to tell anyone, ever. Her parents even had her baptized when she was ten years old and confirmed in 1936 when she was thirteen so she would fit in more easily with her friends and be better able to pass as non-Jewish.

But then her parents wanted her to attend a better school and sent her to the Luisenschule in downtown Munich, a forty-minute street-car ride from their home. At this school the staff knew she was half Jewish as the director and some of the other parents were acquainted with her parents. But by now the Hitler Youth was becoming active, and many political meetings were held at the school. During these meetings her teachers would whisk my mother into a large, dark storage closet while the rest of the children sang Nazi songs just outside. As my mother spoke about this, I imagined her awful fear, locked alone in a dark closet.

My mother stared sadly off into the distance. Then abruptly she said, "We need to stop now. I've got to get dinner ready, and you should do your homework."

"No, no, please go on with the story," I begged.

"I'll tell you more tomorrow."

I couldn't stop thinking of how precarious my mother's situation was, how her survival was dependent upon the discretion of others. Being let in on all of this made me feel close to her, and I could barely wait for the following day to hear more.

On the second afternoon, as my mother poured me a cup of tea, she continued her story. She explained that a few other Jewish children attended the Luisenschule, and as the Nazi movement gained momentum the danger increased for all of them. In addition, she now had trouble commuting to school as Jews were no longer allowed on the streetcar. One day, Ludwig made an appointment with the director of the one Lutheran school in Munich and confided in him their situation. The director told Ludwig, "Of course I'll take her," and he falsified my mother's school papers. Because of this man's help, my mother was able to pass as non-Jewish in that school. The director made up the story that my mother had a heart condition and couldn't perform strenuous activities; that would explain why she wasn't part of the Hitler Youth.

"Every now and then I'd pretend to be weak and grab my chest, like so." My mother demonstrated by dramatically clutching at her heart with both hands. "I had fun doing that." She smiled at the memory.

As the Nazi movement gained momentum, her parents invited friends over to discuss Germany's deteriorating political situation. Her father told her that she could be part of these meetings under the condition that she agreed never to speak a word to anyone about their discussions, including to her best friends. She never knew whom she could trust and whether she'd be discovered. She wasn't able to concentrate at school and thus did very poorly in her studies.

My situation is very different from hers, but we both faked it, I thought to myself. Most people had no idea I was hearing impaired although they may have sensed that I was somehow different. I wondered whether other people might also be hiding something in order to fit in, some way they were different, things about themselves they didn't want others to know. For me, passing meant I had to sacrifice a certain authenticity, had to pretend to be someone I wasn't. Because of my desire to be seen as the same as everyone else and to avoid pity, I wasn't seen in my totality. In my mother's case, though, her very survival was at stake in passing successfully as non-Jewish to the Nazis.

My mother looked drawn and slumped back in her chair. "As the Nazis rose to power, it became too dangerous for Omama to continue performing in the Munich theater. But as our family needed the money, she began teaching acting and diction to students in an upper bedroom in their house. It was very secretive, with the students arriving in the dead of night dressed in dark clothes so they wouldn't draw attention to themselves. Omama had quite a following, and her students always paid her in cash. They knew she was Jewish, and they would recommend her only to other students that could be trusted, but it was still very risky. There was one close call when a student broke down one evening and told Omama that he belonged to the SS and had been told to spy on her. He reassured her that he wouldn't give her away. And he didn't. "This was one of many lucky breaks your omama and I had."

My mother let out a heavy sigh, placed her hands on the table, and stood up.

"But it's time for you to set the table and make a salad," my mother said. "I have to pick up Elliot from chorus rehearsal."

That evening I couldn't stop thinking of my grandmother's students sneaking into her house to learn acting. The risks she took seemed so unlikely for the doting, fussy, cautious grandmother I knew. I wished I could ask her about her wartime experiences, but by now she was quite senile and living in the nearby Jewish Home for the Aged. Omama was no longer the grandmother I knew when I was young, so unfortunately, I'd missed my chance.

The following afternoon my mother again put out a plate of pastries, this time my favorite puffy donuts from Virginia Bakery covered with a thick sugar icing. *Pastries and the Third Reich*, I thought of these sessions that unfolded over the course of the week. A green vase with pink roses, yellow daffodils, and paper whites from the garden perched next to my plate. I was always grateful for these splashes of beauty my mother regularly brought to our household.

I listened enraptured as she continued her story. "In 1937, when I was fourteen, my father started an intense affair with Erika, a beautiful blue-eyed blonde who played the violin and was much younger than he was. Their relationship caused my mother tremendous grief, and I remember many bitter fights between my parents."

She explained that Ludwig often traveled to Berlin to be with Erika, and before long, Erika was pregnant. But Ludwig still didn't want to divorce Omama because he knew that if he did, she and my mother certainly would have been sent to a concentration camp. Omama cried all the time and confided in my mother that she wanted to leave her husband, but that doing so would be simply too dangerous. She was trapped. And because he was married to a Jewish woman, Ludwig couldn't get a job. Omama, through her teaching, earned the money to support Ludwig and also Erika and their new baby daughter, Michaela. Eventually, in 1942, Ludwig moved to Berlin to live with Erika and Michaela and to study to become a Jungian analyst.

"Oh, how painful," I said. "I can only imagine how she felt about her husband leaving her for a younger woman and having a baby with her."

"Yes, she was in deep grief and also scared because Ludwig was now in Berlin and couldn't protect us as much."

"Why couldn't Ludwig get a job?" I asked, confused. "I thought he was a World War I hero and that the Nazis would have left him alone."

"I know, it was strange," my mother answered. "On the one hand, he was a respected German citizen, but he was also married to a Jewish woman, and that put him—and all of us—in a kind of no man's land."

The Nazis had their eye on Omama. Every few months she would receive a summons to appear at the local Nazi headquarters to be questioned. My mother would send a telegram to Ludwig in Berlin, and he'd jump onto the next train to Munich to attend the interview where he could offer his protection as a German husband and recipient of an Iron Cross.

"But every time Omama disappeared into the enormous red brick government building, I didn't know whether she would come out again. I was so afraid for her life. Yet, in addition to Ludwig's Iron Cross, she may have had another protector, perhaps one of her interviewers that admired her theater work. That may explain why, despite being Jewish, she was not sent to a concentration camp."

I set down the donut I'd been eating and remained quiet. My mother's story tugged at my heart and made my quiet hardships of trying to fit in pale in comparison. As I helped her clear the dishes and went to my room to do my homework, I thought, *I can't imagine what it would be like to regularly fear for my mother's life.*

Another afternoon out on the patio, my mother explained how life in Germany changed after the German army's invasion of Stalingrad in the fall of 1942. The Soviets successfully defended Stalingrad, she explained, and they stopped the Germans from advancing farther into the Soviet Union. The Soviets then crushingly defeated the invading German army. With the German retreat from Russia and the Allies landing in Africa and Sicily, it was clear that the war was, finally, turning in favor of the Allies. My mother had felt ambivalent about this reversal; naturally she wanted the Allies to win but at the same time she was in grief about all the Germans she knew that were dying. Every single boy in her Christian Community died on the Russian front, including her boyfriend Kaspar.

In 1942, the Allies began a steady bombing of Munich, which continued until the end of the war. At first Omama and my mother hid in their basement during the air raids, but as it was too flimsy to offer much safety, they'd cross the street and join their neighbors in a solidly built bomb shelter.

"Nobody knew we were Jewish, otherwise we wouldn't have been allowed into the shelter. Omama had been told by Nazi officials that we had to wear the Star of David, but she simply didn't sew the star onto our clothes. People either didn't realize we were Jewish or didn't care. Or maybe because she had a German husband they didn't say anything. We were very lucky."

My mother, now nineteen, was constantly dousing fires in the house caused by the bombs, fixing the blown-out windows, and scavenging for tiles to repair the roof. The streetcar tracks were bombed, so she had to get around on her bicycle. As the streets were filled with shattered glass, her tires were often punctured, which meant she had to search for rubber cement to repair them. And then there were the breadlines; she'd stand in line starting at 4:30 a.m. for four or five hours just for half a loaf of bread and half a pound of spinach. Often, she and her mother ate only a soup made of potato peels. Survival was an exhausting full-time job. I was mesmerized by her stories of her struggles and courage.

After she finished high school, my mother, along with all young Germans, was drafted to do a year of patriotic duty to support the war effort. She was sent to a farm in Bavaria to do some of the heavy farm labor in the fields left behind by the men who were fighting on the front. She was lonely, but the assignment turned out to be a lucky break, as she had more to eat on the farm and could continue to pass, hiding from possible discovery by the Gestapo.

Meanwhile, Omama continued to teach acting, but in 1943, the Gestapo started patrolling her house. Her students no longer came in through the front door but went around to the back garden and climbed in through their bathroom window. Because her lessons continued without the Nazis discovering them, Omama believed she had a guardian angel, perhaps a member of the Gestapo who admired her theater work and was just going through the motions of patrolling the neighborhood because he didn't want to arrest her.

After a year on the farm, my mother returned to Munich where the local Nazis conscripted her to wash the streetcars at the municipal depot. By now, the Nazis were rounding up the remaining Jews to send them off to concentration camps, and my mother was obsessed with figuring out how to keep herself and Omama out of Theresienstadt. First, she planned to pay a guide to take them over the Alps to the border where they'd then make their way into neutral Switzerland.

But that plan fell through when the Nazis discovered the guide's activities and fatally shot him.

My mother and Omama began carrying cyanide pills in their pockets just in case they were deported to Theresienstadt. They'd heard enough rumors by then to know that being sent there was most likely a death sentence. The idea of my mother and grandmother just a pill away from suicide hung heavily on my heart and brought home how dire their circumstances were.

My mother shifted in her chair and leaned forward to pour more tea.

"One morning, out of desperation, I walked next door to share our secret with our Nazi neighbor, Herr Lenner. I thought he might be able to help us in some way. He'd always been friendly to us, but he didn't know that Omama was Jewish. I rang the doorbell, and a maid ushered me into the dining room where I stood awkwardly and watched hungrily as Herr Lenner finished his breakfast of real coffee, milk, cream, marmalade, fresh rolls, cheese, and sausages. Then I went up to him and blurted out the truth, that we were Jewish and that my mother was scheduled to be deported soon to Theresienstadt. I asked whether there was anything that he could do to prevent this. Herr Lenner hissed, 'Those pigs, those swine.'"

She continued, "I thought his outburst meant that he was disgusted by Jews, so I was terrified. But then he said, 'Don't worry darling, I'll take care of it. Go home and stay in your house, and I'll come by later in the evening.'"

At midnight their doorbell rang, and in the black of night my mother could barely make out a beaming Herr Lenner. He gave my mother a warm hug and said, "You don't have to worry anymore; I gave the SS three hundred cigarettes, and they agreed to burn all of your mother's citizen papers." Now, as far as the Nazis were concerned, my grandmother, Anna Ernst Zeise, no longer existed.

My mother reached for her napkin and wiped her eyes. "I couldn't believe that he, a Nazi, would do this for us. I was incredibly relieved, and it renewed my faith in humanity." My mother rarely cried and I sat quietly and took in the significance of what she'd just told me. *If it weren't for the goodness of this Nazi, and other good Germans that helped them, my mother possibly wouldn't exist and I wouldn't either,* I thought. How random and precarious our fates are.

"And, very important," she added, "Omama would still receive our much-needed ration cards, as rationing was handled through a different office. The ration cards didn't allow us much food but did prevent us from actual starvation."

In the final months of the war, Herr Lenner hid my mother and Omama for a few months in his country house in the woods of Bavaria, for even at the very end, the Nazis were still rounding up Jews. He hid other Jews as well. After the war, during the de-Nazification period when the Allies and the new German government were tracking down the worst of the Nazi criminals, Omama wrote a letter on Herr Lenner's behalf, explaining how he had helped them and other Jews to survive. This made it possible for him to escape prosecution as a Nazi war criminal and be reintegrated into post-WWII German society.

The war was finally drawing to a close. In the spring of 1945, the Americans liberated the concentration camp of Dachau and then their tanks rolled victoriously into Munich. At this time Ludwig had returned to living temporarily with Omama and my mother in Munich; even though his mistress Erika was pregnant with his second child, Ludwig still loved his wife and couldn't bear to remain away from her for long. One afternoon Ludwig, Omama, and my mother sat together at the kitchen table and noticed throngs of people walking slowly by their house. They peered out their kitchen window and were horrified by what they saw. The Dachau concentration camp was only fifteen miles north of my grandparents' home, and the Americans had just opened the camp. The surviving camp victims who were physically able walked out of the camp towards Munich, and Omama, my mother, and Ludwig watched in shock as virtual skeletons shuffled along their street in rags and striped pajamas, most of them without shoes. A few knocked on their door and asked for food, any food. My grandparents fed them what they had but soon, they too, ran out of food.

After a few moments of quiet, my mother passed me the pastry plate and asked, "Do you want seconds?" But by then I'd completely lost my appetite. "Then what happened?" I asked.

The survivors walked on to various hospitals, Red Cross stations, and refugee camps set up by the Americans. Although Omama, Ludwig, and my mother had known about the existence of the concentration camps, they'd had no idea how horrific the circumstances were inside; they hadn't yet seen the documentary newsreels that revealed to the world the full extent of the atrocities—the crematoriums, the piles of decomposing bodies, and the hundreds of thousands of starving prisoners.

Omama's three siblings and their spouses all died in Theresienstadt. Their young children had been sent ahead on the Kinder transport to England, and the parents were supposed to follow shortly thereafter, but they didn't make it out of Prague in time. Two of the children, my mother's cousins, made lives for themselves in England, and another cousin emigrated to Palestine.

I knew how terribly Omama grieved the loss of her siblings and the departure of her nephews; she had often shown me their pictures, which were displayed prominently on the little table in her room. Many times, she'd told me stories about their lives. An eddy of grief for her now dragged through my body.

My mother loved the Americans who occupied Munich after the war. She made friends with a few soldiers who, concerned with how thin she was, fed her their rations of canned peaches, Spam, soft white bread, chocolate, and powdered milk. She thrived on the rich food and slowly regained her strength. Through one of the Americans,

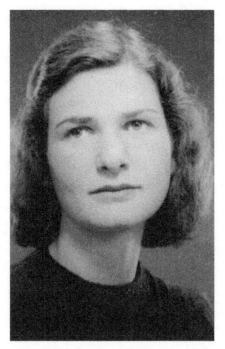

My mother leaving for America, 1947

she obtained a job in a de-Nazification office where the government sought to identify former Nazis, categorize them by how ardent a Nazi each had been, and bring the serious offenders to trial.

I poured myself more tea and added a teaspoon of sugar as she continued her story.

"But by 1947, as hard as I knew it would be to leave my parents behind, I desperately wanted to leave Germany. Much of Munich was destroyed, many of my relatives and friends were dead, and now that it was safe to do so, my parents were finally divorcing. With the help of an American GI, I received an affidavit to come to the United States. When I arrived in New York, I met a German couple who wanted to drive across the country and settle in San Francisco. In exchange for a ride across the country, I took care of their six-month-old baby in the back seat of the car."

My mother stood up, stacked the teacups, and put the sugar, cream, and empty pastry plate onto a tray.

"I loved the drive across the country, but I was a bit frightened at the vast, open space of the Badlands and Nebraska, which were so different from Europe. There was hardly anyone else out on the road. At the end of the trip, when I rode the bus over the San Francisco Bay bridge and saw the Golden Gate bridge and the orange sun setting over the ocean, I knew that this was where I wanted to settle. An acquaintance had given me the contact information for Walter Marseille, who was living in San Francisco, and when I called him, he told me to meet him at Blum's, a popular ice cream parlor. There was an immediate spark between us, and we talked for hours over ice cream sundaes. He then helped me settle into an apartment and found me a job at a nursery school. When I met your father for the second time, he said, 'By the way, you know that I'm going to marry you.' And so it was."[1]

My heart went out to my mother. I had compassion for the real struggles for survival that she went through that I hadn't had to contend with, and that helped put her in perspective for me. I wondered if other children of survivors of the Third Reich experienced similar dynamics of wanting to protect their parents from their own difficulties, but I didn't know any other kids with parents with similar backgrounds that I could share this with. All the kids I knew seemed to have more normal backgrounds. So, in addition to my hearing disability, my mother's dramatic history made me feel different from my peers. Meanwhile, I was grateful she'd told me her story. I felt closer to her than I ever had before, and I hoped for a greater intimacy between us.

Chapter Sixteen

At the beginning of my junior year in high school I met Jim at the home of my mother's friend, Cecily. A talented young violinist, he had just moved to Berkeley from Portland to join the Oakland Symphony, and Cecily invited him to give a house recital to introduce him to her friends and local classical music lovers. When my mother and I arrived at her gracious Spanish Mediterranean home, Cecily took our hands with a smile and ushered us into the large sunken living room, which also served as a music room. Thick wooden beams crisscrossed the high ceilings, and with silent appreciation, I thought the acoustics should be good in there.

There appeared to be about sixty people in the room, all of them at least as old as my mother. All except for me at fifteen and Jim, who looked to be in his mid-twenties. The room went quiet as everyone waited expectantly. Cecily's friend Evelyn, the pianist, sat down at the piano bench and nodded at Jim to begin. He raised his violin to his shoulder, adjusted the handkerchief covering the chinrest, lifted his bow, and launched into a Brahms sonata.

From the first note, I was mesmerized; Jim played with an intensity I hadn't ever seen before. Much of the time he closed his eyes in concentration as his lanky body swayed with the music. His pale face made his dark blue eyes stand out, and locks of blond hair fell over his forehead. By the end of the piece, I was in love. I'd never had this feeling before and was filled with a warm sense of happiness and excitement.

Afterward, as people milled around the buffet on the dining room table, I spotted him talking with a group of middle-aged women who gushed their compliments on his performance. I overcame my usual reserve and went up to him to tell him how much I enjoyed his playing. I was elated when he didn't brush me off and asked, "Do you play an instrument?"

"I play the piano. I'm learning a Mozart sonata for piano and violin."

"Evelyn is from out of town, so I can't work with her. But maybe I could come over to your place and we could try out the sonata," Jim said.

As he spoke my body tingled with an unfamiliar excitement. *This experienced musician wanted me to accompany him?* I marveled. We agreed he'd come over on the following Wednesday afternoon. During our drive home I told my mother about my conversation with Jim, and she smiled happily at me.

A few days later when Jim rapped on our front door, I raced to let him in. He stood on the landing dressed in jeans and a blue shirt that matched his eyes. In one hand he carried his violin in a canvas-covered case and in the other, a leather briefcase filled with sheet music. I couldn't believe this musician was actually in our house.

We started with the Mozart sonata I'd already learned. Immediately my heart soared with pleasure listening to the thick, luscious tones emanating from his violin. Because of my hearing loss, whenever my part included loud bass notes low on the piano, I had trouble separating the violin notes from the piano, but mostly I was able to follow him. Occasionally, he'd gently admonish me, "Slow down," when I sped up, but I gained confidence as we exchanged the melody back and forth between us. I was immensely grateful for my perfect pitch; anytime I found myself lost, I could quickly find my way back by listening to his line and locating it in the score. After we played the Mozart a few times, he rummaged through his bag of music on the sofa, pulled out "Violin Sonata No. 5" (commonly known as "Spring" sonata) by Beethoven and asked, "Are you willing to learn this?" He played the sunny, cheerful theme of the first movement for me, and I was hooked. It was technically too difficult for me to sight read, but I agreed to work on it, along with a charming sonata by Schubert. The pleasure and confidence I gained from our playing together made me think that maybe I could become a professional accompanist.

For the next few months, Jim came over once a week, without fail, to play music with me. While other teenagers were dating and partying, I practiced the piano, and I loved it. I wanted to make it worth Jim's while to play with me. Occasionally, we talked about things other than music—my school, his family and friends back in Portland, and the music he was learning for the symphony. He was twenty-four, he told me. He was so much more interesting than the boys in high school. By now I was fantasizing that he might become my boyfriend, but I worried that our nine-year age difference would be a barrier to a relationship beyond making music together. I suspected he hadn't guessed I wore hearing aids, and I was too timid to tell him. I wanted him to know, but I was afraid he would be less interested in me as a musician if he knew I had a hearing disability.

One afternoon after playing for an hour, we decided to take a break from the Beethoven sonata and moved over to the sofa near the piano. Jim sat close to me and rested his arm along the back of the sofa near my shoulders. My mother was out shopping for groceries, and at last I could sit with him alone. After a few minutes, he scooted right against me. As I talked, he looked at me intently and with a thundering heart, I thought, *Oh my God, it's actually going to happen, he's going to kiss me!* I stopped talking and time seemed to slow down.

His eyes moved from mine down to my mouth, and he leaned in close. Then he put his hands over my ears and drew my head toward his, his lips moving in closer and closer to mine. But then from my ears came a horrible screech that made Jim jerk backward in shock. His touching my hearing aids had set off their awful shrill feedback, and we were both jolted out of the moment. Mortified, I blurted out that I wore hearing aids and that he'd set off the feedback whistle. He nodded but didn't say anything and I looked up at him again, hoping he'd lean in again for a kiss, but he just sat there, studying me. After a long pause, he stood, picked up his violin, and said, "Let's play the Schubert sonata." The moment had passed and I was crushed.

One afternoon a few weeks later, Jim invited me to go with him to hear a regional competition of piano concertos. It was down to the semifinals, and the piano soloists were to be accompanied by the Oakland Symphony, of which Jim was a member. I was surprised my mother let me go out with Jim and Michael, a friend of Jim's who had a car. She could be strict, but she was supportive of anything having to do with classical music, and I knew she was pleased Jim was in my life. My heart swelled with happiness that Jim wanted me there; clearly he liked me. As I sat next to Michael that evening in the audience listening to the pianists thundering through their concertos, I only had eyes for Jim, dressed in white shirt and black slacks, accompanying the soloists in the second violin section of the orchestra. Afterward, Michael drove us back to my house, and Jim and I got out of the car. Jim led me up the pathway toward the front door, took my hand, and guided me under a tree. He put his arms around me, drew me to him, and, careful not to touch my ears, leaned down and gave me a gentle kiss on the lips. A tide of happiness rippled through my body. I watched him make his way back down to the car and then floated back to my room in a trance. *Maybe I could be his girlfriend,* I fantasized. *What's a gap of a few years?* It was a week before my sixteenth birthday, and I couldn't have asked for a better present.

We continued to play music together for the next few months with me working hard to learn new pieces. We engaged in a musical conversation, weaving the melody as a web between us. Occasionally we shared a kiss, and each time the thrill of it vibrated through my body. I wondered if he would ever ask me out on a real date. At the same time, I couldn't quite envision what a date with him would entail. Was I really ready for that?

As the heavy winter rains finally gave way to a luxuriant spring, we sat one afternoon on the patio eating pastries with my mother. Jim told us he had just been offered a job as the assistant conductor at the Sun Valley Dance and Music Camp in Idaho for the summer and suggested I apply. I desperately wanted to go. I fantasized about having time alone with Jim to maybe see movies or go out for ice cream, and I wanted to be with other kids who shared a love of classical music.

The ten-week camp was expensive, so my mother agreed to let me go on the condition that I write to my father in Germany and ask if he'd pay for it. I hated writing to him for money; I wished my mother would do it, but we both knew that he was more likely to agree to pay if the request came from me. He had come through for me a few times in the past, paying once for new hearing aids and later for part of the airfare for my trip to Germany. I suspected he would approve of my attending a music camp, and over the next several weeks I anxiously awaited his reply. Finally, a thin blue airmail letter arrived in the mailbox with his familiar handwriting in fountain pen. I dashed to my room and tore open the letter. He wrote, *I'll split the amount with your mother; now that she's remarried, I don't see why I should have to pay all of it.* I knew that for years he'd paid virtually no child support, and his cheapness upset me. Over dinner that evening I told my mother and John what my father had written. John insisted that they would manage somehow, and that I should definitely go. My heart overflowed with gratitude.

The music camp was sponsoring a competition for prospective piano students to play a piano concerto with the camp orchestra at the end of the summer. The auditions would be held early on at the camp. My piano teacher thought I should enter the competition and suggested I learn Mozart's "Piano Concerto No. 23 in A Major." So, in addition to the pieces I was working on with Jim, I dove into trying to master the concerto. I loved the piece, it fit my joyful mood that spring. The first and third movements are exuberantly cheerful, the slow movement beautifully expressive and poignant. I knew it was a long shot for me to win the competition; there were many older and finer piano students from around the country who'd be auditioning. But I didn't mind the experience of learning the concerto, and I decided to be realistic and not get my hopes up about the audition.

I vowed to have a different camp experience than I'd had in Germany, so when I arrived in my dorm room and we were all settling in, I overcame my usual reluctance and forced myself to tell my three bunkmates that I was hard of hearing. I went on to explain why I wouldn't be able to participate in the discussions in the dark at night. They smiled and said, "That's cool."

On the second day, Laurel, a voluptuous girl with long ash-colored hair, plunked herself on her stomach on the bunk above me and, peering down from her mattress, asked, "Do you want to go out for an ice cream?" She was a year older than I and was studying voice. She included me whenever she went out with her friends and we quickly became close.

The camp was made up of large wooden buildings nestled on a school campus in the outskirts of Sun Valley. The area was surrounded by tall mountains, pine trees, and lush meadows. Every morning I woke up and took in the beauty of the tall mountain peaks from our dormitory room. During the day I was happily engaged in my daily classes of music theory, chamber music, music history, chorus, and ballet. In my private piano lessons, I learned new pieces by Bartok and Schubert while perfecting my Mozart concerto. After class I'd go join other kids for ice cream and walks around the campus. I was making new friends.

But I rarely saw Jim. Sometimes I spotted him on the other side of the campus surrounded by a group of older students; he would nod and smile at me but made no attempt to come over and talk. Occasionally I passed him in the hallways in the company of a pretty brunette. With a stab of pain, I wondered if our connection was over.

Regardless of how much I loved music, one thing became clear to me that summer: Due to my hearing loss, my becoming a professional musician was out of the question. There was fierce competition from other pianists, but worse, I realized that my limited hearing was going to make performing music at a professional level impossible. When I played solo piano, I couldn't discriminate well between the various low notes, so I compensated by learning the fingering and playing the notes correctly. It seemed my determination was enough to get me past that issue. But accompanying other musicians, where I had to clearly hear their part, was another story.

One afternoon in my chamber music class, I was paired up to play with a cellist, and as we tackled the slow movement of a Beethoven sonata, I soon realized I couldn't discriminate the low notes of the cello over the bass notes of the piano. Violin was easier for me to play along with because its range didn't extend down into the low range of the piano, which was harder for me to discern. Additional instruments just added to the muddle of sound. To my chagrin I had to tell the cellist and the teacher that I simply couldn't hear the cello part. The realization that I couldn't be a professional accompanist stung, but at the same time I felt freed. As I let go of my fantasy of being a musician, I could almost feel the burden of that goal lifting off my shoulders. To compensate for my disability, I'd worked incredibly hard, meticulously learning the fingering and memorizing as much as possible. Until that moment of surrender, I hadn't realized how hard I'd been working to accompany Jim.

I saw Jim only at our chorus rehearsals of Mozart's "Requiem in D minor," which the whole camp was learning for the end of camp performance. My heart soared with the music of the mass, but to my distress, I couldn't hear myself among the other voices in the chorus, so out of fear of singing seriously off tune, I mostly just moved my lips. Sometimes Jim's blue eyes twinkled at me from across the rehearsal room, but he made no further effort to engage with me.

Then one morning at breakfast, Julie, one of my bunkmates, not knowing of my interest in Jim, said, "Did you know that Jim is going out with Karen?" My gut sank. I knew she was one of the camp's ballet dancers and I wondered if she was the girl I'd seen walking with him in the hallways. As the others chattered on about this piece of news, I remained silent. *Didn't what we had count for anything?* I'd been aware all along that our nine-year age difference was probably a barrier to a romantic relationship. And even though I tried to push these thoughts out of my mind, I couldn't help thinking that he, at age twenty-four, probably shouldn't be kissing a sixteen-year-old. Yet I yearned for some kind of connection with him.

The competition to perform the piano concerto was a few days later. From backstage where I stood huddled with the other contestants, I watched the conductor's face closely so I'd be able to lipread him when he called out my name. When he finally did, I edged my way onstage under the lights to the gleaming black Steinway Grand near the conductor's podium. I was happy to spot Jim sitting in the dark at the back of the auditorium; he was one of the judges, and his presence reassured me. I smiled, but he didn't smile back, and in that moment I realized that he no longer had any interest in me. My stomach felt weak, but I tried to put the thought aside and concentrate on the concerto.

Although I knew the piece, I'd been practicing it all those months in relative quiet; I wasn't prepared to play it in the midst of a roaring orchestra, and I quickly lost my place. The conductor told me to start over, but it was hopeless. I simply couldn't follow the orchestra. After two more brief tries, the conductor said, "Enough! Next!" and another pianist stepped out and took my place. My cheeks flushed with mortification, particularly because Jim had witnessed how abysmally I had bombed. But it was also a relief. There were just some things that my hearing disability made impossible for me to do well. Maybe it was time I stopped putting myself in those difficult situations.

I looked over to where Jim was sitting, but he was whispering animatedly with a pretty brunette who appeared to be in her early twenties. I realized in a flash she must be Karen. The way they leaned into each other, and the sight of his arm draped over her shoulder, hurt more than my failed audition.

After the camp ended, I didn't hear from Jim again. I was so miserable that once I was home, I stopped playing the piano altogether. Between the loss of Jim and my realization that I couldn't be a professional musician, I didn't have the heart to touch my beloved instrument for the next several years. But I was relieved to have the stress of trying so hard behind me and I threw myself into my schoolwork. I confided in my mother about Jim and Karen, and she murmured sympathetically, although she also pointed out that he was too much older for a real relationship. I also told her how I struggled during the audition with the orchestra, which surprised her. She had no idea how difficult accompanying musicians could be with a hearing loss. Finally, I told her that my studies had become more demanding, so I wouldn't have the time to practice the piano, and although disappointed, she accepted that. I associated the ending of my first love with the ending of playing the piano. For the time being, both love and the piano would be put aside.

Chapter Seventeen

To my relief, my last year of high school was great fun. I developed friendships with two sisters from Munich whose family was on sabbatical in Berkeley, and I enjoyed my classes tremendously, particularly modern dance and English, where we immersed ourselves in the English classics.

That year I also took an important step in my quest to be more open and honest about my hearing loss. My extracurricular Shakespeare class was taught by Mr. Lawrence, an elderly British gentleman with a scraggly mustache and a pronounced accent, who played LP records of famous English performances of Hamlet, Macbeth, and King Lear. He insisted we close our eyes and listen to Shakespeare's language. With no text to refer to and no lips to read, I'd absolutely no idea what was being said. And, because of his mumbles through his mustache, I couldn't understand him as he guided the class in discussions. I was so afraid of being left behind and getting a low grade that I finally plucked my courage and told him after class one day that I was very hard of hearing, that I depended on lipreading, and that it would be really helpful if I could follow along with the text.

"But you look so normal," he said.

I was stunned. *What did he think a person with hearing loss should look like?* I thought. But at the same time, I felt a wave of relief that I'd finally spoken up for myself and that I'd have the text to read. *I need to do this more,* I thought. This marked the gradual beginning of my coming out as a person who was hard of hearing.

One day in my history class, my classmate, Ross, stood up and announced he was leaving high school early to join the Israeli army. The Six Day War had recently ended, and Israel needed more young soldiers to defend the country. "Come and join me," he said. I was impressed. Compared to my classmates, his sense of purpose at only age eighteen made him seem like a man. His older sister, he told us, was traveling with him to work on a kibbutz in southern Israel near Egypt to help defend the border.

"What's a kibbutz?" I asked, and he explained that it was a social experiment, a collective whereby all the income earned by the members was shared equally. Children were raised and educated together, and, although they spent time with their parents in the afternoons and evenings, they slept separately in sleeping quarters devoted entirely to the children, watched over in shifts by different kibbutz members. I was intrigued.

The more I thought about life at a kibbutz, the more excited I became. I would be only seventeen when I graduated, so I thought about taking a year off before college and traveling to a kibbutz to work. I wondered if spending time at a kibbutz could help me feel connected to my Jewish roots. I remembered my grandmother telling me about her beloved siblings' death in the Theresienstadt concentration camp, and I had been profoundly affected by my mother's account of surviving the Nazi regime in Munich. I hadn't been raised in the Jewish faith, but I was deeply moved by their stories. I wondered if I could be genuinely Jewish if I hadn't been raised religious. Maybe I could find the answer at a kibbutz. When I told my mother I wanted to go to Israel, she was very supportive, as she often was of my endeavors. "We'll figure out a way to get you there," she said.

My mother had a German acquaintance, Nina Chermoni, who had emigrated after WWII from Germany to Israel. She lived at the Ayelet HaShahar kibbutz in the Golan Heights near the Lebanese border, and upon my mother's suggestion, I wrote to her. Nina quickly replied with a warm invitation to come and work as a volunteer at the kibbutz.

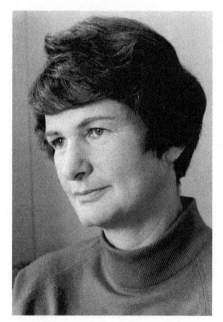

My mother, 1968; photo credit: Ernst Anman

Meanwhile, my mother and John would spend the year in Zurich and in Oxford for John's sabbatical. Like me, my mother was very excited about the upcoming year for she would be returning to Germany for the first time in twenty-two years. I was very happy that she would finally see her close friends again and would also see Elliot, who one year earlier had left to attend an international boarding school in the Swiss Alps. I decided I'd visit my father and the Stolzes in Munich on my way to Israel; it had been three years since I had seen them last, and I counted the days until I would see them again.

The spring before I left for the kibbutz was tinged with poignancy; after a series of strokes, my beloved Omama had finally died in the Jewish Home for the Aged. In some ways I had lost her years earlier. She'd suffered from dementia for some time, so my sorrow was mixed with relief that she wouldn't be left alone in Berkeley while we were all in Europe. I was sad to have Omama, a source of unconditional

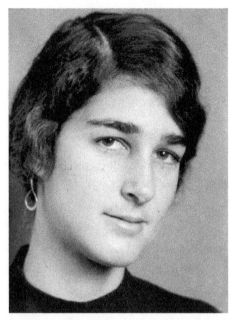

Off to Israel; photo credit: Ernst Anman

love and kindness in my childhood, simply fade out of my life as we all busily prepared for our year in Europe, but I was excited about my plans for the future. Despite mourning my grandmother's death, my life was opening up, and I couldn't wait for high school to end.

That August I arrived in Munich on my way to Israel and was lovingly folded back into the Stolzes' family circle. Over the next two months, in addition to spending time with the Stolzes, I studied German at the Goethe Institute and took classes in ceramics where I learned to throw pots on the wheel. I loved the creativity of shaping concrete forms from amorphous blobs of wet clay. Twice a week my father picked me up for visits at his apartment and leisurely strolls in the Englischer Garten. I enjoyed my time with him more than when I'd seen him three years earlier; as he aged, he'd become softer and less abrasive. He still didn't ask much about my life, but he spoke less about German politics and the Russians, and when he saw me, his eyes would light up with delight and he would envelop me in big hugs.

The afternoon before I left for Israel, we sat in his living room for tea and a plum tart we bought at the corner pastry shop. My father interrupted our game of chess and placed a thick folder next to me on his round coffee table.

"These are the deeds to Schloss Bischofstein (Bishop's Stone castle). That's where I grew up in in East Germany," he said, handing me a black and white postcard of a baronial manor house built in 1705 perched on top of a hill in a forest.

"If East Germany were ever to be reunited with West Germany and I'm no longer alive, you and Elliot should file a claim to get the property back. It belongs to us even though it's now in Russian territory."

I'd rarely heard him talk about his childhood growing up in Schloss Bischofstein overlooking the village of Lengenfeld-unter-dem Stein and knew virtually nothing about his family.

"How'd you get this property?" I asked. "And what happened to it since you left Germany?"

My father went on to explain that his father, my grandfather, Gustav Marseille, was descended from French Protestants called Huguenots. They'd fled religious persecution by the Catholics in Marseille, France, several hundred years earlier, and, like many other Huguenots, moved north into Germany. Gustav was an educator and wanted to start his own school. In 1901, he bought the hunting lodge built on top of a small hill deep in the Thuringian Forest in what later became East Germany, the area where the Brothers Grimm had collected their fairy tales. Gustav converted the dilapidated lodge into an international boys' boarding school where he could apply his many progressive pedagogical ideas. As a child growing up there, my father had the special position of being the eldest son of the principal of the school.

"In the afternoons, we boys had fun exploring in the hills behind the school where stones from the remains of a twelfth-century fort were scattered everywhere. The school was grand and had a spacious inner courtyard which was surrounded by gardens, red clay tennis courts, and gentle, rolling agricultural land and woods. We played games in the meadow while the adults took their afternoon tea nearby on the terrace surrounded by lush gardens. It was pretty idyllic." My father smiled wistfully down at the floor at the memory and my heart soared hearing about this romantic part of my heritage.

The school was not far from Weimar, home to Goethe and Schiller, leading figures of the German Enlightenment 150 years earlier. My father placed his teacup on the coffee table, stood up, and started pacing animatedly across the floor. "You know, inside the building was a small ballroom where Gustav, your grandfather, who was a great lover of classical music, hosted musical events and dances. Gustav was an excellent cellist and often performed in a string quartet. You would have loved your grandfather." Instinctively I knew that was true, and I was sorry I never got to know him.

I took a second helping of plum tart and added a generous dollop of whipped cream. The possibility of our ever gaining access to this property within East Germany seemed very remote, but I delighted at my father's recounting of his early picturesque years.

"But then Schloss Bischofstein became the site of tremendous loss for me." He spoke in a flat voice and stared out the window onto the linden trees lining the street below.

"When I was six years old, my mother gave birth to her third son, and soon after she was hospitalized in an institution. She was diagnosed as bipolar back in 1907, but it is possible she suffered a bad case of what we now know as postpartum depression."

Regardless, while she was at the institution, she managed to hire a stagecoach, kidnap my father and his two younger brothers, and disappear deep into the Thuringian Forest with her three boys for two days until the police finally found them.

"Were you scared?" I asked.

"I don't remember much. But after that, my poor mother was sent to a locked ward, and I was told that she'd died. That was just devastating. Soon my father married our governess. Gustav hoped in this way to provide a mother for us three boys, but I never liked my stepmother. We never bonded, and she became attached to my infant brother Wolfgang, who essentially became her own child."

Was my grandmother truly crazy? I wondered. *Or was she a woman locked and silenced so my grandfather could marry the governess? Why couldn't she be cared for at home? Did my father inherit his dark, erratic moods from her? What, if anything, did I inherit from her?* It frustrated me that I'd never know the truth.

"Nine years after Gustav's remarriage, we three boys came down with scarlet fever, and Wolfgang died. He was only nine, the youngest. A year later, when I was sixteen and on a school excursion to a nearby lake, I was sailing with my other brother, Ernst. A freak storm arose, the boom slammed into the side of Ernst's head and the boat tipped over. Ernst was a good swimmer, but he was knocked unconscious by the boom and drowned while I tried to save him. That was a terrible time for me and my father," he said matter-of-factly.

I thought about how horrific it would be to lose Elliot that way. How would I ever get over that kind of pain? "That's just horrible," I said.

"Yes, it was," my father said. "I dove down repeatedly to try and grab him, but he was beyond my reach. Then a year later Germany lost WWI and the country went into deep mourning. You've no idea how completely demoralizing it was for the Germans, losing the Great War. Then in 1918 my father died in the Great Flu epidemic. He was a wonderful, warm, and generous man; everyone loved him." My father paused. "But the worst was yet to come when I was a student in Marburg."

My father walked slowly into the kitchen to put on water for more tea. *The worst was yet to come?* While I waited I tried to imagine what could be worse. "Go on," I said when he returned to the living room.

"One day I bumped into an old peasant woman from the village near Schloss Bischofstein. She told me that my mother, your grandmother, was not dead, after all, but had been living all these years in an asylum, not far away. I immediately set off to find her, but it was too late. She had died just six months before."

I was stunned; I'd had no idea my father had lost his mother this way. I didn't know that he'd been through any of these tragedies. What tremendous grief to have to deal with at such a young age—so much loss. This was the first I'd ever heard about my paternal grandmother, and my heart hurt for my father, for her, my uncles, for all of them. I was also surprised by his speaking to me so personally, it was the first time he had done so. I was finally beginning to see what contributed to his becoming such a difficult person.

"Then what did you do?"

He described how he went to study in Marburg and earned a PhD in philosophy under Martin Heidegger. While in Marburg, he became friends with Hannah Arendt, the philosopher and journalist who later reported on the trial of Adolf Eichmann in Jerusalem in 1961 and became famous for her writings about the banality of evil. My father reminded me of her visit in Berkeley in 1955 when she was a visiting professor at the university.

"One evening when she was at our house—you couldn't have been older than four years—you served her hors d'oeuvres of nuts, olives, and coconut strips."

I had a hazy memory of her dark, piercing presence.

My father continued with his story. In 1932, after breaking off contact with Heidegger because Heidegger refused to condemn Nazism, my father moved to Vienna to train to be a psychoanalyst. He met and corresponded with Anna Freud, Sigmund Freud's youngest child, who'd followed her father into the field of psychoanalysis. Later my father moved to Berlin and trained under the psychoanalyst Siegfried Bernfeld, but then became involved in an underground resistance movement against the Nazis. As he was in danger of being arrested because of his activities, he decided to emigrate to America.

Was he a spy? I wondered. I wanted to know exactly what my father did in this underground organization, but I didn't want to interrupt his story.

"I had no money to pay for my ship passage, so I struck a deal with the ship's officials. In the summer of 1937, your clever daddy invented and published the rules for a five-suit bridge game which included a fifth suit of green leaves. This set off a fad for five-suited decks, which lasted through 1938. I managed to persuade the ship's officials that I was seeking a patent for this invention, that I'd make a lot of money and would share a portion of the profits with them. To my great relief they let me on board the boat without charging me for my passage. However, at the dock in New York, I was met by a man who was waving his own patent for a five-suited bridge game that he managed to obtain before me. That was the end of that financial venture, but I managed to slip into the anonymous world of New York City and never did pay for that ocean crossing." He smiled at the memory.

"After World War II, Schloss Bischofstein fell into the Russian zone and was converted to a local communist headquarter. Which is the situation now."

He stood up, ready to clear the dishes from the coffee table. I didn't want the conversation to end, but, without saying a word, I helped him stack the dishes on a tray. Slowly he carried the tray into the kitchen.

My father looked exhausted and gray. The dark, sunken circles under his eyes appeared particularly prominent. He walked back into the living room, picked up the folder, and stored it in a cabinet in his bookshelf. I'd so many more questions to ask, but he said, "It's late. I'll take you back to the Stolzes."

As my father drove me through the leafy suburbs of Munich, I thought about the story he had just told me. I had always sensed in him a stern, haunted loneliness that he covered with bluster and pre-occupations. Maybe because of my own periodic loneliness as a child, I'd always been pained in the presence of his loneliness, his separate-ness. And now I had a better understanding of the history that had shaped him and made him emotionally inconsistent, the tragedies that must have tormented him. *My God,* I thought. *By the time my father was seventeen years old, his entire family was dead.*

Years later, after my father's death and after the Berlin Wall came down, Elliot and I, with the assistance of attorneys, unsuccessfully tried to regain possession of Schloss Bischofstein. Sadly, due to complex bureaucratic maneuvers and regulations by the German government with jurisdiction over properties in former East Germany, our family's property was kept out of our hands. Losing this part of my father's legacy was painful and served as another reminder of the difficulty of receiving something truly positive from him.

Chapter Eighteen

As the bus jostled along the road towards Kiryat Shmona near the Golan Heights in northern Israel, I scrutinized the map spread across my knees. Boarding the bus in Haifa earlier that morning, I'd asked the driver, "Ayelet HaShahar?" He'd nodded. Now, two hours later, I was beginning to worry that he'd forget to let me off at the kibbutz. With my finger on the map, I traced the names of the hamlets we were passing; some of the signs were in English as well as Hebrew so I could track the bus's progress. Looking out the window I didn't see any buildings that might belong to a kibbutz, only lush orange orchards and agricultural land.

Finally, I spotted a sign for the Bronze Age archaeological site, Tel Hazor, which from the map I saw was on the other side of the highway from the kibbutz. Nina Chermoni, in her letter inviting to me to stay, had suggested I read James Michener's 1965 novel, *The Source*, loosely based on Tel Hazor. Her letter mentioned that the famous archaeologist Yigael Yadin had excavated Tel Hazor in the 1950s and had returned a year ago, in 1968, for his last season on the dig. "If you like, in your free time, you can join some of the other volunteers from the kibbutz for the final stages of the dig." I had romantic fantasies that I would find some major artifacts of an ancient civilization.

I shuffled down the aisle to the driver, who looked up at me and nodded. Then the brakes screeched, and the driver hopped out and hauled my large suitcase from inside the luggage compartment and dropped it next to a crooked hand-painted sign that read, *Ayelet HaShahar*. Without a word, he jumped back onto the bus, which took off leaving behind a plume of black fumes. I looked at the sign, its faded red arrow pointing toward a narrow path through the orange trees.

I was wearing brown shorts and a blue and white checkered short-sleeved shirt, sneakers, and a navy blue bandana around my neck. I thought it would be hot in the Israeli countryside, but in January in the foothills of the Golan Heights it was surprisingly chilly.

As I lugged my heavy suitcase along the path, I was thrilled at the sight of the brilliant ripe oranges popping against the glistening snow-capped mountains of southern Lebanon. The scent of the citrus trees drifted heavily through the air and all was silent as I passed through the orchards. I was excited about my new life on the kibbutz. I hoped to find out if this experience would make me feel more Jewish. And even more important, I was ready to present a new version of myself to the world. I would make sure these people didn't view me as a shy bookworm. I would show them a carefree, spontaneous, outgoing young woman. I not only wouldn't keep my hearing loss a secret, I'd go out of my way to tell people about it and ask them to face me when they spoke. "I am hard of hearing," I'd say. "I need you to look at me when you talk." This was new territory for me, and as the path meandered through the swaying trees my body trembled.

After twenty minutes I came to a wider path where I saw a group of elderly women walking together, chattering amongst themselves. I asked for directions and they pointed me towards the kibbutz office, a small wooden bungalow, where I met Nina, a short, plump middle-aged woman who welcomed me with a warm smile. In broken English she offered me coffee from a large thermos. Part of her job, she explained, was to supervise the volunteers who came to work at the kibbutz.

She led the way along the lush garden paths lined by lemon bushes and magenta bougainvillea, past the dining room set back on a large lawn, past the small bungalow residences belonging to couples and individual kibbutzniks, and finally, past the covered swimming pool and the chicken coop to a cluster of dark wooden cottages, which she explained were the sleeping quarters of the volunteers. Colorful laundry hung on clotheslines surrounding the cottages, and three young men pulled hoes through a large vegetable patch nearby. Other men were lounging in canvas slingback chairs sipping from mugs on the front deck of one of the cottages. Two of the cabins were reserved for female volunteers, Nina explained, and she motioned for me to step into the larger one. The room had eight bunk beds along one wall and rickety dressers on the opposite side. Worn paperbacks lined a bookshelf made of cinder blocks and pine boards. Nina introduced me to Elizabeth, a volunteer from Zurich, who was seated at an old desk writing a letter. Nina asked Elizabeth to show me around and then told me to stop by the office at 6:00 the next morning to receive my job assignment and work clothes.

Elizabeth was in her mid-twenties, I guessed. She was tall and thin, and her thick brown braids were pinned across the top of her head. She had round rosy cheeks and a kind smile, and I liked her immediately. As I quickly changed into jeans and a sweater she told me, in excellent English, that she and her fiancée, Hans, had been working at the kibbutz for the past three months. I was pleasantly surprised to discover that people spoke English here.

"It's been our dream to take off for a year after our university studies and travel around the world before settling down to get married and find jobs and have children," she said. "We want to travel now because I'm not sure when we'll ever have the chance again. We just love it here. And we've already stayed two months longer than planned."

Elizabeth explained that the kibbutz usually housed up to twenty volunteers, mostly from Europe but that at the moment there were only ten.

"Right now, you and I are the only two female volunteers. I am so happy to have another woman around," Elizabeth said.

She linked her arm into mine and walked me next door to the men's cabin to introduce me to Hans, who was stocky, jovial, and as friendly as Elizabeth. I also met Andrew from London, aristocratic, fair-skinned with curly blond hair, and dark-haired Luciano from Milan. Their friend Gaston, from Luxembourg, was living in the small one-person cabin behind ours.

"He's very nice but he's cleaning out the chicken coop now. You'll meet him later," Elizabeth said.

I wondered why Elizabeth didn't share living quarters with Hans. As if she'd read my mind, she said, "I won't sleep with Hans until we are married." I was surprised. *If he were my fiancée, I probably would sleep with him,* I thought.

Because the volunteers came from all over Europe, their common language was English. And because English wasn't their first language, they spoke more slowly and simply, which made it easier for me to understand them. And in keeping with my resolution to be more forthcoming about my hearing limitations, I explained to each of them that I loved that they spoke English slowly because I could understand them better. I lifted my hair up above my ears and showed them my hearing aids. To my relief, they just nodded matter-of-factly.

Later that afternoon Elizabeth and I took a walk in the fields of the kibbutz.

"Ayelet HaShahar means morning star in Hebrew," Elizabeth explained. "It was first settled in 1915 by immigrants from Europe."

As we ambled in the orange groves, she pointed out the major landmark in the field, the half-buried remains of a Syrian plane shot down in 1948. I was curious about this as my understanding of Israeli history was vague.

"What happened in 1948?" I asked.

"I don't really understand that much myself, it's complicated. But in 1948 Israelis fought against the surrounding Arab countries that tried to capture Palestinian territory that had been ruled by the British. In Israel the 1948 war is now known as the War of Independence. In the north Syria and Lebanon fought against Israeli forces, and that's how this plane ended up here. During this war thousands of Palestinian Arabs were forced out to other Palestinian territories that were captured by Egypt or Jordan or other Arab states. And many of them were sent to refugee camps and are still there today."

I had so many questions, but Elizabeth wanted to tell me more about the kibbutz. Ayelet HaShahar, like most kibbutzim, was self-sustaining and self-governing, and their profits were shared equally among all the members. Most of their money was made from agriculture, mainly the orange and apple orchards, honey, and the fish from the ponds, as well as from the guest house where visitors paid to stay. Kibbutz members made decisions about day-to-day life together at regular council meetings. Some members with special expertise, such as accounting, kept the same job for years, while others rotated among different jobs. Currently there were over eight hundred kibbutz members, mostly Ashkenazi Jews from Russia and Germany who had either escaped to Palestine before the war or survived the Holocaust and then made their way to Israel.

"And, as you probably know, another war broke out between Israel and the surrounding Arab countries in 1967, and during the night, even though it's been eighteen months since that war ended, you can still hear shelling between the Syrian and Israeli forces on the Golan Heights just a few miles away. But you'll get used to the noise," she said. She went on to explain that the young children went to a group daycare from 7 a.m. to 4 p.m., then, as they grew older, they attended a grammar school at the kibbutz. At fourteen, the teenagers were housed together apart from their parents.

"The whole kibbutz is like one giant family; I think it's quite wonderful," Elizabeth gushed.

"Where are the young Israeli men and women? What do they do

after high school?" I had hopes of meeting a handsome Israeli sabra (a native-born Israeli), perhaps a hero from the 1967 war.

She said, "Oh, they aren't at the kibbutz, they're all doing their military service, both the men and the women. You'll see them only when they come back for the holidays or sometimes when on leave for Shabbat dinner at the kibbutz."

I had forgotten about the compulsory military duty for all young Israelis. Years later I read that after being exposed to the larger world of Israel, and especially the vibrant cities like Tel Aviv, many of the young members didn't want to come back and live the simpler agricultural life of the kibbutz. Enticing young adults to stay at the kibbutz was a problem throughout Israel and it wasn't clear that the kibbutz experiment would ultimately survive.

That evening Elizabeth and Hans escorted me through the gardens to the dining room, where most of the kibbutzniks ate with members of their family and close friends. Elizabeth, Hans, and I sat down with our trays of lamb stew, steamed vegetables, olives, yogurt, and pita bread at a table designated for the volunteers near the large windows that overlooked the lawn where children played tag. I looked around and was struck by the easy camaraderie and animated conversations taking place at every table. Although trying to hear in a noisy dining room was always a challenge and reminded me of the cafeterias in my elementary and high school, I quickly realized that it would be easier here eating with the volunteers because they spoke English so simply. *I'm going to like it here,* I thought.

While we were eating our dessert of halva, a tall young man with blond hair and a cropped reddish beard bounded over to our table, hugged Elizabeth, shook hands with Hans, and then plopped down in the empty chair next to me.

"This is Gaston; he's been here for nine months. He has the cabin behind ours," Elizabeth said.

Gaston turned to me and when I saw his blue eyes lock with

curiosity onto mine, I knew with an intuitive flash that I'd fall for him. He was, I guessed, in his late twenties. He spoke English slowly and clearly, and as with Elizabeth and Hans, I had no trouble understanding him.

"What work do you do at the kibbutz?" I asked.

"I've done different jobs," he told me. "I've plowed and fertilized the fields with a tractor, picked oranges and apples, worked in the metal shop repairing agricultural tools, and now I'm in charge of feeding the chickens, cleaning out their coop, and collecting the eggs."

I hung onto his every word but wondered what would make an adult man leave home to do manual labor at a kibbutz for an extended period. Gaston, Elizabeth, and Hans weren't Jewish, but they all seemed drawn to the dream of kibbutz life, of socialist ideals, and a life of physical work in nature.

"What did you do in Luxembourg?"

"I taught math in a high school, but I've always wanted to travel. So, I quit my job and here I am. I love it here."

With that he stood up and said, "Let's all take a walk."

The four of us left the dining room and talked as we strolled the kibbutz paths. Then, as we approached our cabins, Elizabeth said, "I have to get up early to work the breakfast shift in the kitchen, so I should get to bed."

Reluctantly, I said I should probably get to bed too, as I had to meet Nina early in the morning for my job assignment.

Gaston squeezed my hand and said, "Goodnight, see you tomorrow." My entire body thrilled with pleasure.

Back in the cabin, continuing with my resolution, I explained to Elizabeth that I slept without hearing aids, which meant I couldn't hear an alarm clock. "Could you shake me awake in the morning?" I asked.

"Ja, but it'll be very early, because I have to be in the dining room at five to help prepare breakfast."

That did seem very early, but I didn't want to risk oversleeping, especially on my first morning. "I don't mind," I said.

Suddenly I heard a deep rumble off in the distance. "It can't be thundering," I said. "It's been such a clear day."

"Oh, that is the shelling between the Israelis and Syrians in the Golan Heights. You'll hear them most nights but don't worry, the Israelis won't let the Syrians get any closer," Elizabeth said.

I felt a little nervous being that close to a war zone, but Elizabeth seemed pretty nonchalant about it. I said goodnight, took off my hearing aids, and slipped under the covers into my bunk bed. Without my hearing aids I no longer heard the small explosions. Lying under two heavy wool army blankets, I happily reviewed the events of the day, wondered what my work assignment would be, and fell asleep fantasizing about Gaston kissing me.

After a breakfast of hardboiled eggs, hummus, fish, raita, olives, and tabbouleh, I made my way to the kibbutz office.

"Your first assignment is to work in the laundry room washing and ironing sheets," Nina said. "But before you start, let's get you some work clothes."

I was disappointed. Doing laundry didn't sound very exciting; I'd rather have been assigned to plowing the fields, but I knew that it wouldn't be long before I'd be rotated to another job, and I wanted to be helpful and cooperative in my new home away from home. "Sounds great," I said with a smile.

We ambled over to a bungalow that stored used clothing for use by the volunteers. Pants and shirts hung on a long rack and used boots of different sizes perched on the shelves. I chose two pairs of khaki shorts, a pair of brown work pants, two long-sleeved blue shirts, and a pair of sturdy work boots. Now I'd look like a proper kibbutznik. I wished my family and friends at home could see me like this.

Nina dropped me off at a low-slung building with one large room bathed in steam and lined with washing machines, dryers, and large roller presses for ironing sheets. Several stout middle-aged women bustled about, lifting baskets of laundry as a radio played music in the background. Magda from Poland showed me how to operate the washing machines and feed the damp sheets through the fat rollers to press and dry them. Working the rollers required two people, one to position the sheet between the rollers—Magda made clear how to be careful not to get one's fingers caught—and the other to receive the sheet as it came out at the opposite side of the roller. Then two people worked together to fold the sheets.

At the beginning of each hour, everyone would stop work for five minutes and listen to the news summary on the radio while sipping coffee from thermoses. The women explained that practically everyone in Israel listened to the news several times a day; one never knew what might happen next. I couldn't understand a word as it was in Hebrew, and without being able to lipread, I wouldn't have understood even if it had been in English. I worked in silence as the women chattered in Hebrew, but I didn't mind not being part of the conversation; it felt good just to be part of this kindly group. At eleven o'clock we stopped an hour for lunch, then at three o'clock I was told that my workday was over. I had the rest of the day off and could do what I liked. The job wasn't exciting, but the seven hours whipped by fast. And I was excited about seeing Gaston again over dinner.

The next few weeks melted into an idyllic blur. I ate all my meals with Gaston and the other volunteers. The weather gradually warmed, and soon the pool was open for swimming. I usually opted out of swimming because being in the water meant I'd have to take my hearing aids off, which meant I couldn't be part of any conversations. Instead, I spent the afternoons sunbathing on the lawn surrounding the pool, hoeing and weeding in Nina's little garden in front of her bungalow, and taking walks in the fields with Elizabeth, Hans, Gaston, Luciano, and Andrew. Andrew was preparing to apply to graduate school in London in Middle Eastern affairs and was in Israel to learn more about the history and politics of the area. I enjoyed listening to him as he talked of his plans to become a foreign diplomat. Luciano was out to have a good time and would grab my waist and try to kiss my hand or my cheek, which I thoroughly enjoyed. I noticed that Gaston became stiff and silent when Luciano flirted with me.

Over the next several weeks I spent more and more of my time alone with Gaston, taking walks or talking over coffee on his deck. The kibbutz had a music bungalow with a small grand piano that a kibbutznik, Helga, from Belgium, had brought in a few years earlier. Some of the children took lessons from her and practiced after school in the music room, but usually they gave up after a couple of years, so the piano didn't get much use. Although it had been over a year since I had played the piano, I wanted to show off for Gaston. One evening I flipped through the music inside the piano bench and found some Schubert impromptus and Mozart sonatas. I played some of the pieces I was familiar with while Gaston sat in a chair and watched me. It was warm, so he flung open the windows and door and I could see the stars beaming at me off in the distance. Soon, to my surprise, several of the elderly European women carried folding chairs out to the little patio outside the music room to listen. Some of them brought their knitting while others, eyes closed, nodded their heads in time with the music.

"The music is bringing back memories of their childhoods in Europe," Gaston said.

I was elated that I could contribute to the kibbutzniks in this way; it was an easy way for me to make people happy.

The next day I went to Helga to ask if she could lend me more piano music so I could give my little audience more variety. Helga had a beautiful Blüthner grand piano that practically filled her whole bungalow. Generally, the kibbutz, which encouraged egalitarianism, frowned upon people owning luxury items, but she was a profession-ally trained pianist who'd married a kibbutznik. They wanted her to be happy at the kibbutz and so they made an exception by allowing her to bring her piano.

"So many of the older people here are homesick for Europe, despite the atrocities that happened there," she said.

During the rest of my stay, I practiced and played for an hour several evenings a week in the music room and my little audience on the patio grew. Gaston was always present at these little recitals. Sometimes he brought out the guitar stored in the closet of the music room and sang songs to us in French. He had a rich baritone voice, and I loved the way he looked over at me shyly while he played. I couldn't take my eyes off the glistening golden hairs on his forearms. Members of our little audience nodded sweetly at us as we played, and my heart was happy.

Chapter Nineteen

One afternoon while we were eating a picnic lunch on the big lawn by the dining room, Gaston asked me, "How would you like to go with me to Tel Hazor? Yigael Yadin is winding down the dig there, but I hear they need volunteers to help with the final work. It's just across the road."

"Oh yes, let's go!" I gushed.

A few days earlier Nina had pointed out the bungalow that James Michener had lived in for a few weeks while conducting research for his book *The Source*. I had loved his novel, a sweeping history of the Jewish people which followed a stone age family through to the present day, all situated around a mythical tell (a small hill).

Years later in 2005, Tel Hazor was awarded a World Heritage designation by UNESCO as a site having cultural and historical significance worthy of preservation and protection. After our picnic, Gaston and I walked the twenty minutes through the kibbutz apple orchards and crossed the narrow highway onto the site. I looked around at the low labyrinthine walls of bleached yellow stone and at a large flat dirt platform lined with rectangular pillars. At the center of the site, an open-sided metal shed with a corrugated tin roof protected the workers from the hot sun. Ten volunteers sifted dirt through fine mesh screens, which reminded me of sifting flour for a cake. The burly young site supervisor came bounding out of the shed, pumped our hands, and introduced himself as Ben. "Oh, I'm glad you've come," he said. "We could use some help."

Ben assigned me the job of carrying buckets of dirt to the crew of sifters. He nodded towards a clay floor nearby that was sectioned off with string into a one-meter grid. Several buckets of dirt stood within each of the one-meter squares; they all needed to be carried to the shed and sifted. Ben said that when that was done, I could help with the screens. Gaston's job was to number the pot shards and enter them into a registry book.

I was fascinated by Ben's recounting of Tel Hazor's history. He told us that in the Middle Bronze Age, about 1750 BC, Hazor was the largest fortified city in the area and very important within the Fertile Crescent. Hazor had trading ties with Babylon and Syria from whom they imported tin to make bronze. Now Mr. Yadin was finishing up the dig at the Canaanite layer dating from approximately 1500 BC, and they were looking for any small artifacts like beads, potsherds, or small coins. Ben pointed out the low-walled remains of the 1000 BC Israelite village lower down the hill. He said that all the larger and dramatic artifacts had already been found and carted away, but the small remains were invaluable in assigning dates to different sections and layers of the site.

Ben made us feel very welcome. Mostly we all worked in silence, which suited me fine. I didn't have to look up to make the effort to lipread as I sorted through the remains of clay and dirt clods in my screen. I liked being included so easily as part of a team.

Gaston and I began spending a couple of hours a day at the site after finishing our work at the kibbutz. Every day we carried buckets, sifted through dirt, and catalogued potshards. Gaston always pulled his folding table and chair over to where I was working so we could be near each other. As I shook my mesh screen, I periodically gazed at the cobalt blue sky, taking in the beauty of the view. Beyond the yellow walls of the site rose the green foothills of the Golan Heights, and in the background glimmered Lebanon's Mt. Hermon, still covered with snow. I couldn't have been happier.

Gaston and I spent more and more of our free time together, working at Tel Hazor, playing music, and talking for hours on the quiet deck of his cabin. One evening, six weeks into my stay at the kibbutz, Gaston suggested that on our next day off we visit the city of Safed, about a forty-minute bus ride south of Ayelet HaShahar. Safed, he explained, was an important center of Kabbalah and Jewish mysticism and had a wonderfully preserved medieval quarter. I was elated at the prospect of a day off the kibbutz alone with Gaston, and I was eager to see more of Israel.

A few days later we rode the bus to Safed, perched high on a rocky outcrop. On the way, as we looked out at the beautiful Sea of Galilee below us, surrounded by green hills and red poppies, I wondered if this was how it looked when Jesus practiced his ministry. In Safed, I was transported back to biblical times as we watched Orthodox Jews with long beards and side curls ambling through the maze of stone alleyways in the medieval part of town.

On the ride back to the kibbutz, the bus was very crowded, and Gaston and I stood pressed against each other and the other passengers. As the bus lurched around a sharp corner, he wrapped his arm protectively around my shoulders, then leaned down and kissed me on the lips. A tug within my body pulled me towards him, and I wanted him to kiss me again. He held me close to him for the rest of the ride.

That kiss quickly broke down any remaining barriers between us and soon we became lovers. Ten years older, tender, and patient, he was a gentle teacher, and, liberated from the introverted bookworm self of my high school years, I plunged wholeheartedly into my first love affair. I was surprised at how easy and natural my first sexual experience was, and each time we made love I gained confidence and my sexual attraction to him grew. I felt myself blossom in this relationship with a man who could hardly keep his hands off me. I was relieved that my hearing disability had clearly not prevented me from attracting a man and I could hardly wait to write about my first affair to Ann back in Berkeley. I spent more and more time in Gaston's cabin, sometimes overnight.

Soon Elizabeth figured out what was going on.

"I can't believe you're sleeping with him before you're married," she said sharply.

I was upset at her reaction and at the same time felt slightly guilty.

"We're in love. I don't see what could possibly be wrong with sleeping together," I answered. Elizabeth turned on her heels and walked away without another word.

I continued to enjoy my time in Gaston's cabin. Anything that felt this good and made me this happy couldn't be a bad thing, I told myself. But to my sadness, my friendship with Elizabeth grew strained and soon she and Hans left the kibbutz to return to Switzerland. As nothing could be kept a secret at the kibbutz, before long the other volunteers and Nina found out about my relationship with Gaston, but I was relieved that nobody else seemed to care. I even confided to my mother in a letter about my love affair, and she wrote back that she was very happy for me that I had a boyfriend. I was impressed by her open mindedness and appreciated being able to share this with her.

But soon after we started to sleep together, I discovered to my dismay that Gaston had major mood swings. If another volunteer flirted with me, Gaston wouldn't speak to me or anyone else for the evening, then the next morning he'd be cheerful again as if nothing had happened. I was careful not to incite his jealousy, but the slightest greeting I gave to another man could result in Gaston's cutting me off again until the following day. I was also bothered that he had no plans for his future. He wasn't sure how long he would remain at the kibbutz or what he would do afterwards. I loved life at the kibbutz, but I knew that eventually I would leave; I wanted to go to college and live in a larger world than the kibbutz could offer. One evening, as we lay in bed entwined in each other's arms, I told Gaston my plans for college. He withdrew his arms and turned his back to me for the remainder of the night. As always, when he rejected me this way, I was hurt.

Several times I tried to tell him how bothered I was by his withdrawals.

"It is really hard for me when you don't talk to me about your feelings," I would say. But it was to no avail as he wasn't capable of a conversation about it.

Over the next few months, we made several short trips to Jerusalem, Bethlehem, Nazareth, Ramallah, and Hebron. Gaston was always in a better mood when we traveled, which I assumed was because it was just the two of us and he had my undivided attention. We timed our Jerusalem trip to coincide with the annual Israeli Independence Day parade in late April. There had been a huge turnout for the parade the previous year (1968), with over half a million people watching as soldiers marched through the recently united Jerusalem, and as military planes flew overhead displaying Israel's military might. That year's parade drew international condemnation for being too provocative to the Arabs.

The 1969 parade was a more low-key undertaking. It began with several different pre-Independence Day marches through various villages in the West Bank and ended in Jerusalem. Gaston and I, along with soldiers, civilians from around the country, and kibbutzniks, marched for three days from Ramallah in the West Bank. We civilians were directed to the center aisle and the soldiers marched on either side of us, automatic rifles slung over their shoulders. I felt uneasy as we marched through Ramallah with hundreds of armed Israeli soldiers while Palestinian civilians peered out at us from the windows of their small stone dwellings or looked up from their ploughed fields. A group of children in flip-flops with rocks in their hands ran after us, but the women called them back, anxious not to provoke an incident.

It didn't seem right to me that the Israeli army was marching through land that had once belonged to the Palestinians, but when I voiced my concerns to Gaston, to my surprise, he took Israel's side.

"The Arabs have to pay the price for invading Israel. And they keep saying they want to push the Israelis into the sea."

I believed it was more complicated than that. I was troubled by the fact that Israel was occupying lands that Palestinians had lived in for centuries, and that so many Palestinians had been displaced from their homes. But I didn't want to get into a discussion with him about this because I knew it would just lead to a disagreement. Gaston, I was learning, was politically more conservative than I was, and this difference between us greatly bothered me. Although I was deeply drawn to the beauty, history, and antiquity of the land, I was increasingly disturbed by what I saw as Israel's discriminatory treatment of the Palestinians. And even though I was Jewish by blood, I wasn't raised Jewish by my assimilated Jewish mother. While I loved being part of kibbutz life and their Jewish celebrations, I wasn't drawn to taking on the Jewish faith. I was becoming clearer about my Jewish identity. *Maybe I can be Jewish by blood, but not in actual practice*, I thought.

Each night of the march, the Israeli army set up hundreds of tents, outhouses, and food stations in huge campsites in the fields outside of Jerusalem. The first night, as I looked across all the campfires twinkling in the field below me and the stars shining above, I imagined we were a medieval army on the move. On the third day we marched into Jerusalem, and I was enchanted by its ancient golden walls that seemed to welcome us. We spent the next two days wandering around the colorful bazaars of old East Jerusalem, and I was blissfully transported into the past as we visited the holy sites—the Temple Mount and Dome of the Rock, the Wailing Wall, the Mount of Olives, and the Church of the Holy Sepulcher. We hiked along the Via Dolorosa, the path Jesus is said to have carried his cross from his sentencing by Pontius Pilate to Golgotha where he was crucified. It seemed unreal to

be actually walking in a place described in the Bible. The narrow cob-
blestone road wasn't lined with olive trees as depicted in the hymns,
but rather with hundreds of tourists and souvenir shops. Yet there was
a silent reverence among us all as we solemnly walked along the Via
Dolorosa.

After we left Jerusalem, Gaston and I took a bus to the southern
port and resort town of Eilat on the northern tip of the Red Sea. The
surrounding desert was barren and bleak. It was May, but already the
temperature was in the low 100s, and in the blazing heat I felt as if I
were dissolving into the surreal lunar landscape. We swam early in the
mornings, and as soon as we stepped out of the water the dry wind
evaporated the moisture, leaving a salty crust on our bodies. In the
afternoons we melted into lovemaking and tried to cool off beneath
the rotary ceiling fan in our room. At night, after a simple dinner of
falafel, hummus, and olives at a sidewalk café, we scoured the town
for its popular coffee with vanilla ice cream. As were alone together,
Gaston was in good spirits, and I was happy in the presence of his
warm and easygoing side. For the time being I was able to forget his
oppressive possessiveness, and I didn't want this time to end.

After a few days it was time to return to the kibbutz. On the way
home we decided to stop in the Gaza strip, which had been captured
from Egypt by Israel only two years earlier. As soon as we stepped
off the bus and into the baking hot parking lot, I noticed we were the
only non-Arab people on the street. Men in black and white kaffiyehs
gathered and stared hard at us. One young man rushed at us waving
his arms and yelling in Arabic. It was clear that Israelis and foreigners
weren't welcome.

"This is creepy. Let's get out of here," I said.

Before Gaston could answer, something sharp smacked against
my cheek. Gaston raised his arms to defend himself against a shower
of stones being hurled at him by a group of teenage boys surrounding
us on three sides. Adults stood watching grimly, arms crossed, but

no one made a move to stop the boys. Gaston grabbed my arm and dragged me back into the bus station. He examined my face and said, "You're bleeding." He dabbed my cheek with his handkerchief. Gaston was bleeding from lacerations on his upper arms and one on his neck. We sat, shaken, on a couple of metal chairs close to the ticket office as the ticket master watched in silence while we washed our cuts with water from Gaston's thermos. My hands trembled at what a close call we'd had. We could easily have been more badly hurt. We caught the next bus out of Gaza several hours later and arrived with relief back at the kibbutz. Once again, I realized how complicated the relationship was between Israelis and Palestinians. There was a lot I didn't understand.

Upon our return, I asked Nina if she could assign me to a different job than working in the laundry room. First, she gave me the task of weeding and watering the vegetable gardens. I enjoyed the physical work as I hoed the dirt and hauled wheelbarrows full of weeds and debris to the dump behind the dining hall. After a month of hoeing, she switched me to a job in the kitchen peeling potatoes, carrots, and onions for eight hundred people's daily meals. Kibbutz life had made me quite strong, and I could hoist heavy burlap sacks of potatoes into the large machines that spun around and cut off most of the peels. Then I dumped the potatoes and carrots into big tubs of water, and with a knife, sliced off any bits of skin the machine had missed. I peeled the onions by hand, and soon my hands were stained yellow from the juice. Although the job was repetitive, and I worked mostly alone, I didn't mind. The work was meditative and offered a break from the strain of trying keep up with conversations. In between onion tears, I looked out at the irrigated green kibbutz fields, the Golan Heights, and Mt. Hermon—a view I couldn't get enough of. But when the dig at Tel Hazor wound down for the summer because of the sweltering white heat, I started thinking of returning to Berkeley. Andrew and Luciano had left for further travels in the Middle East and Europe. I missed their companionship, even more so as Gaston's mood swings continued to strain our relationship.

One afternoon, as Gaston and I walked over to the bungalow that served as the kibbutz post office, I was handed a thick letter from the University of California at Berkeley. I'd told Gaston a few months earlier that I was interested in studying anthropology and archaeology, and my hands shook as I tore open the envelope.

"I've been accepted to the university!" I told Gaston, waving the letter in the air.

Without a word, he turned from me and stomped away. Over the next few days, he became more withdrawn than ever, and we had less and less to say to each other.

"What do you want to do next in your life?" I would ask him, and he always gave the same answer: "I don't know. I guess I'll stay here for now." I was distressed by his lack of initiative.

Late one afternoon I decided to plant a row of sunflowers in the little garden in front Nina's cottage. She was stretched thin with administrative tasks in the main office and was always appreciative when I worked her plot of land. After I finished hand-watering the fledgling stalks and was about to return to my cabin, Nina stepped out onto her deck holding two mugs of steaming hot coffee. I marveled again at how the Israelis could drink such quantities of hot coffee and tea, always insisting that the hot drinks made their skin feel cool by comparison.

"Come and sit with me," Nina said. "I've something I want to talk with you about."

She looked serious as she placed the mugs down on the table and motioned for me to sit next to her on the wooden bench. I was nervous. Maybe she was bothered by my sleeping in Gaston's cabin, although the kibbutzniks seemed easygoing and pretty much ignored what the volunteers did during their time off. But she was from my mother's generation, and she might not approve.

"We discussed you at our all-kibbutz council meeting last night. We came to a unanimous decision."

I could feel my face flush and perspiration beading on my forehead.

Nina looked at me and put her hand on top of mine. "We all really like you. You're a hard worker, and we decided we'd like you to stay here and become a permanent member of the kibbutz." She went on, "Also, you are Jewish, so you belong here in Israel. What do you think about joining us?"

I was stunned but relieved. I blurted, "My grandmother was Jewish, but my mother's only half Jewish and I wasn't raised Jewish."

"If your grandmother was Jewish that makes your mother and you Jewish," she said, smiling. "You belong here with us."

It felt good to be wanted and I was momentarily tempted to answer with a grateful yes. I wondered, *if I weren't Jewish, would the kibbutz council still extend this offer?* But their offer wasn't going to change my decision to return home and start my higher education.

"I love it here so much, everything about this kibbutz. Everyone is so kind and generous. I've thought a lot about staying here longer but ultimately I belong back in California. It will be very hard to leave but I want to return home to start college this fall," I told her.

She sighed. "Yes, I was afraid that would be your answer."

That evening I told Gaston about my conversation with Nina. The date for my departure was coming up and our separation was imminent. We were finally talking about it.

"If you cared about me, you'd stay with me here at the kibbutz," he said.

I felt terrible, but I steeled myself.

"I'm only eighteen. I'm not ready to make a long-term commitment.

I don't want to hurt you, but I want to go back to the States and go to college." I didn't tell him that I was no longer sure I loved him.

"Yes, you're young." Gaston sighed. "Go on back to America if that's what you want, maybe that's best." I was wounded; I felt I was being dismissed too easily. But I was also relieved. During my time at the kibbutz and in my relationship with Gaston, I had blossomed. It was one of the few times I'd ever felt a sense of belonging in a group. I'd had the opportunity to work on an archaeological dig. I'd even become clearer about what being Jewish meant to me—I could identify as Jewish by blood without being religious. But I was ready to start college.

My last two weeks with Gaston were strained as it was clear we were biding our time to our inevitable goodbye. Our lovemaking was tainted with a quiet melancholy. But in the end, he resigned himself to my departure and saw me off at the Tel Aviv airport. A bittersweet sorrow passed through my body, and I cried as he enveloped me in a final hug. I knew I would miss him and the kibbutz.

After my return to California, Gaston and I wrote letters for a few months while he stayed on at the kibbutz. Finally in one letter I tried to explain as best I could the cultural and political revolution of the late '60s that was sweeping Berkeley, but he never wrote back. Maybe he just couldn't relate to the world I was now inhabiting, or perhaps he had simply moved on. I was sad about the end of my first love relationship, but I knew I'd made the right decision. I was ready to move on to the next phase of my life.

Chapter Twenty

In the fall of 1969, I was living off campus in Barrington Hall, a co-op dorm where students worked part time to offset their rent. It was a wild time to be going to UC Berkeley. I was surrounded by hippies in tie-dyed T-shirts and the smell of marijuana. Telegraph Avenue was crowded with vendors selling handmade jewelry, crystals, and macramé holders for hanging flowerpots. The campus hadn't yet settled down from the People's Park riots, where police opened fire on protesters who had gathered to save a community garden from being destroyed to build more UC Berkeley dormitories. Students were regularly demonstrating in Sproul Plaza against the Vietnam War. Many of my dorm mates, in between trips to the library and carrying out their required jobs for the co-op, spent much of their time either making out or tripping on psychedelics.

Margaret, an anthropology major a year ahead of me, was a perfect roommate for me—reserved but friendly. We soon realized that we had archaeology and international travel in common, and surrounded as we were by students taking drugs, we knew there was one important thing we had to do to initiate ourselves into life at Berkeley: We had to try marijuana. Over the course of several evenings, we perched nervously on the edge of our beds and encouraged each other between coughs to inhale deeply, but neither of us felt any effect. Finally, late one night, we started giggling hysterically about absolutely nothing. Time slowed down, and I felt euphoric. I was acutely aware of the colors and the lights in the room, and I had trouble following a train of thought. We knew it had happened; we were stoned. After getting high a few more times, I felt fully indoctrinated into Berkeley culture. I was ready to plunge into my classes.

I majored in anthropology, and in my freshman year I took classes on the politics of the Middle East. I had dreamy memories of Israel and wanted to learn more about its history, so I decided I would eventually apply to the junior year abroad program at the Hebrew University in Jerusalem.

The large lecture classrooms at UC Berkeley worked well with my hearing disability. I would grab a seat in the front row so I could understand the professor. But, as usual, I had more trouble in the smaller classes where there were discussions, for I had trouble following who was speaking. In the small sections I told the teaching assistants about my hearing loss, but that still didn't make a difference in my being able to follow the class discussions and I was left out. But, as most of my classes were large lecture classes and I diligently studied the textbooks, I did well in my courses.

At the kibbutz, I'd become more comfortable telling new friends about my hearing disability, so at college, I began with Margaret, explaining why I couldn't talk with her at night in the dark. But the noisy meals in the dining room and the frequent parties with loud music continued to cause me difficulty and pain. I often left the dining room after I finished eating, missing out on the socializing. At parties, I'd either stand on the outskirts quietly observing, or, if someone approached me, I'd do the best I could with lipreading. Even when I told others I was hard of hearing, that admission didn't necessarily help my situation. I still couldn't hear them above the cacophony of noise that was common in university life. Sometimes I tried to control the conversation by asking lots of questions; that way, I wouldn't have to try and understand random questions addressed to me. By setting up the context, I could more easily figure out the answers.

But it wasn't only at parties or in the dining room where I struggled. Because of my hearing disability, I simply didn't fully comprehend the full import of some of the momentous national events that were happening at that time. In April 1970 President Nixon expanded the Vietnam War by ordering combat troops to invade Cambodia. At Kent State University that May, four students peacefully protesting against the war were fatally shot by National Guard troops. The Berkeley campus broke out in riots with violent confrontations with the police, but I didn't know why. Barrington Hall was abuzz with agitated discussions and the news was playing on the television full time, but as usual with big group conversations and the television, I couldn't make out what was being said. Yet again I felt left out, and now I didn't have the tolerance for feeling excluded as I had in my younger years, so I was more upset. Fortunately, I could resort to reading the newspaper to enlighten me, but this always put me a day or two behind my peers. Once I comprehended the full extent of the upheavals, I was shocked and dismayed, and over the next year, I periodically demonstrated with other students against the war.

In the summer after my freshman year. Margaret and I worked together on an archaeological dig in Arizona and then moved into a two-bedroom apartment with two friends. The four of us lived companionably together, dividing our time between studying, dating, hanging out with each other, demonstrating against the war, and lying on the floor listening endlessly to Simon & Garfunkel's song, "The Sound of Silence." As usual, without being able to lipread I couldn't understand the lyrics to the music my peers so easily listened to, and I relied on reading them, when available, to figure out what was being said. Music was such an important part of the culture at the time, and this inability to easily follow the lyrics on records and the radio or at concerts was an even greater source of frustration to me than it was back in high school.

But fortuitously, I discovered photography. I took a photojournalism class and fell in love with it immediately as photography relied on my visual skills. I spent many happy hours in the journalism department's darkroom watching my images magically rise up to meet me as I bent over the developer tray. With photography, I started to feel like an artist.

During this time, I regularly visited my family home in the Berkeley Hills and spent wonderful evenings with my mother, John, and Monica, now four years old. I was gratified to see my mother so happy since her marriage to John and her developing career as a therapist. With her painful past largely behind her, she was relaxed and sweet with me, and we had reached a welcome and easy rapport with many long companionable conversations over tea. Monica would throw her arms around me when I came to visit, and I loved playing with her and her dolls and stuffed animals. It was refreshing to periodically escape the wildness of Berkeley campus life and enjoy some easy, quality family time. But I missed Elliot, who was now attending St. John's college in Santa Fe.

One evening at a Berkeley party, I spotted a young man, tall and slim with dark brown hair and warm hazel eyes that sparkled behind his glasses. Elegantly dressed in a red cashmere sweater and new brown slacks, he was refreshingly different from the guys I was used to seeing on campus, with their long hair, beards, and hippy clothes. The host told me that Michael, age twenty-six, the son of a British lord, had just finished his PhD at Oxford and was working at a lab on campus completing his two-year post-doctoral fellowship in biochemistry. Michael was only six years older than I, but he had an air of worldly weariness that made him seem like an old soul. He stood at the edge of the room sipping wine, regally aloof. My first impression was that he was a bit arrogant, but when he glanced over at me and then strode towards me, my heart pounded.

"Good evening, how are you?" he asked, with a pronounced Oxford English accent. "My name is Michael."

I burst into laughter at his formality and his accent.

"You've got to be kidding! Is that accent for real?"

"It is indeed."

"Do you know anybody here?"

"No. I've just arrived in the US. How are you enjoying the party?" he asked.

I chattered on while he smiled. Occasionally he interjected, "Quite, quite."

At the end of the evening, he asked me to accompany him to an Ingmar Bergman movie the next night. I happily replied yes and was even happier when I found out that it was a foreign film that would have subtitles. That night I left the party in a daze. Michael seemed to be from another world than I was inhabiting, and I was flattered that a son of a British lord was interested in me.

We started going out several times a week, and early on I told him about my hearing disability. He was interested, asking me about both the logistical and emotional aspects of my hearing loss, and for the first time I shared deeply with another person the full impact my hearing loss had had on my life. Despite his accent, I understood him well because he articulated so clearly. He was kind and understanding, which drew me close to him.

With great enthusiasm, Michael introduced me to more foreign films, classical music, and fine art, and over the following months we attended many concerts and museum exhibits. He was taking my cultural education in hand, and I relished it. Michael described how he had accompanied his father to various ceremonies and functions at the House of Lords and how, at the annual opening of Parliament, he and other sons of lords had sat at a designated spot near the queen. But, he clarified, his father wasn't a hereditary peer; rather, he was a created peer, which meant that upon his father's death, the peerage would not be passed down to Michael but would expire. His father had founded the National Marriage Guidance Council in England, and as a result, the English government had awarded him a lifetime peerage.

Despite his air of aristocracy, Michael hadn't grown up with money; his parents were working-class Labour Party activists. He spent his early years in a dilapidated apartment building next to a pile of rubble remaining from the German bombing of London during World War II. He told me that his parents owned a thatched roof cottage in the beautiful Cotswolds near Oxford.

"How did your parents get the money to buy it?" I asked.

"One afternoon, when I was six years old, I was digging a hole in the patch of dirt behind our apartment. I found what looked like interesting rocks with scribbles on them and I filled my bucket with them. I'll never forget the stunned look on my mother's face when I emptied the bucket upside down and all the rocks clattered onto our metal kitchen table."

"What were they?"

"They were old coins from hundreds of years ago, possibly from a pirate's booty. I'd literally dug up a treasure chest."

His parents wanted to keep the discovery a secret because they feared the coins would be taken from them and given to the queen's treasury, as was usually the case of discovered caches from that period. So, over the next few years, they drove to different antique shops throughout England and sold one coin at a time. No one asked questions about just one coin, and gradually his parents saved enough money to afford to buy a house and send Michael and his brother to private school.

"Wow. It's like a fairy tale," I said.

Soon I was spending most nights at Michael's apartment. I tried to ignore the fact that while my friends were intrigued by Michael, they found him aloof. He was kind to me but was formal with most everyone else. Although he had many acquaintances, he had only one friend back in England.

"Doesn't it bother you, having so few friends?" I asked.

"Not at all, I don't need friends," he replied.

That troubled me. There was something familiar about him, and then I realized he reminded me of my father and his contradictions—his warmth and passionate intensity alternating with a haughty remoteness.

In the meantime, I'd been accepted to the junior year abroad program at the Hebrew University. I was looking forward to studying politics and anthropology in Jerusalem. Many of the classes in my program would be taught in English, but we were required to have a "working" knowledge of Hebrew. My program advisor had suggested I study for ten weeks that summer near Jerusalem at an Ulpan, an intensive Hebrew language program. I also thought, since I had reservations about Michael this early in the relationship, this would be a good time to split up with him. Despite my love for him and the pleasure I took in our many shared interests, a gut instinct told me that I shouldn't commit to him, that he was too rigid, too difficult, too much like my father. But the thought of breaking up and losing his warm support of me was distressing. I was deeply torn. Michael, too, was upset about my imminent departure. We both cried when we parted at the airport.

As soon as I started the Ulpan summer program, I realized how much Hebrew the other twenty participants in my program already knew. They'd been raised in the Jewish faith and had learned at least the rudiments of the language from Hebrew classes growing up, whereas I didn't even know the alphabet. After the first week of the Ulpan, I was already hopelessly behind, desperately trying to make sense of the guttural sounds made in the back of the throat that were impossible to lipread.

By the third week, I realized that once again I'd underestimated the impact of my disability, especially on learning a foreign language. The class was moving much too rapidly, and learning and understanding a foreign language, as I already knew from my attempts to learn German, was extremely difficult. Also, my advisor hadn't spelled out for me, nor had I read the fine print of the program description, that while many of the classes in the English department were taught in English, most of the other classes were in Hebrew. Halfway through the summer, after I failed yet another quiz, I realized to my distress I'd have to drop out of the junior year abroad program. *I need to be more realistic about my limitations*, I thought, yet again. *I can't keep getting into situations that are over my head. It's just too painful.*

On the way back to Berkeley with my tail between my legs, I decided to stop in Munich to visit my father whom I hadn't seen for two years. He suggested we spend a week together in Innsbruck in the Tyrolean Alps of Austria. At first I was delighted, but then, to my dismay, I saw that he had packed his suitcase with dominoes, chess, and Go for us to play. My heart was no longer in these games. I could also barely tolerate his continual rants about German and Munich university politics and I was distracted by my aborted year abroad and doubts about whether or not I should get back together with Michael.

Michael had been sending me imploring letters, begging me to return to him in Berkeley, and the letters were making me anxious because I was conflicted about whether to get back together with him. I wanted to drag my father away from his games, to confide in him and ask his advice, but I believed my personal life was too complicated to explain and that having so many similarities to Michael, he wouldn't understand my reservations.

However, one morning I managed to persuade him to leave the dark hotel room and take a hike with me in the nearby alpine mountains. We found a lovely steep trail through a lush green meadow dotted with wildflowers, but I was disturbed that he insisted on ponderously stepping backwards up the trail with deep and strenuous squats, sweat streaming down his face. I remembered how, when I was a child, he used to do this as I accompanied him on walks up the steep Marin Avenue in Berkeley.

"This will strengthen my calf muscles for skiing this winter," he said.

"You look weird. Do you really need to do this?" I asked. "It's slowing us down, and everyone's looking at us. Can't you just enjoy the hike like everyone else?"

"I don't care what everyone else thinks. This is important. It is good for my calf muscles." Once again, I was upset by his stubborn unwillingness to adhere to regular social norms and his insensitivity to my feelings.

That evening, I decided to cut short my visit with my father and booked a flight to Berkeley. Soon, I was back in Michael's comforting arms, but I felt ambivalent. I welcomed the security of being back with him, yet I couldn't dispel my reservations about his social reserve and arrogance, the ways he was like my father.

Not long after my return, I noticed that my mother, John, and several of their friends were walking around and smiling mysteriously saying that they had "gotten it." While I'd been away that summer, they had taken est, the Erhard Seminar Training, a program recently founded by the charismatic salesman, Werner Erhard. The program consisted of a two weekend, 60-hour self-help program that was part of the "human potential movement" that encouraged its participants to take responsibility for the outcomes in their lives. Everyone strongly urged me to take est and I was curious. I thought it might help me find clarity about whether I should stay with Michael. And Michael, not wanting to be left out, signed up to take the training with me.

During the training, I was swept up into the power of positive thinking. Philip and I could just "decide" to make our relationship work. Flush in the afterglow of the two weekends of immersive training, Michael and I decided to get married as soon as I graduated from college. Also because of the training, he made another big personal decision: He would switch from his career path as a biochemist to become a medieval art historian. When Michael was growing up, his father had insisted he become a scientist or a doctor, and he'd dutifully followed his father's wishes. But Michael had always been passionate about medieval art history, not science. Now that he'd been swept up in the 1970s Berkeley "follow your bliss" mantra, he was fired up to go after his own dreams, and he persuaded me to move to London after our wedding so that he could enter the master's program specializing in medieval art history at the Courtauld Institute of Art, essentially throwing away his Oxford PhD and post-doctoral training. I was supportive of him following his lifelong dream.

As soon as I graduated from college, we had a lovely small wedding surrounded by friends in my mother and John's garden in Berkeley. Then we began taking steps to move to England. For me, the decision was complicated. I knew I would miss Berkeley and my family, particularly as my mother and I had been getting along well over the past few years. And I would miss Monica, too, now eight years old. But I focused my thoughts on the adventure of living in London. My mother and John had generously given me $1,000 to buy a piano, and I looked forward to taking lessons again. And we had a place to move to—Michael's brother was moving out of his suburban apartment in north London and suggested we take over the lease.

Four days after we arrived, Michael handed me the phone; someone from Germany was trying to reach me, but to my dismay I discovered I couldn't hear a thing, only the electrical buzz of the telecoil produced by my hearing aid and silence in the receiver. The telecoil that had made it somewhat possible for me to hear on the phone in Berkeley didn't work at all with the English phone system.

With frustration I thrust the phone back at Michael. The caller was my father's attorney who informed Michael that my father had died earlier that day of a sudden heart attack. To my surprise I went numb and couldn't cry.

The next day, Michael and I took the overnight ferry and train to Munich. We were met at the hospital morgue by the funeral director who sat us down at a table in his office, placing a thick binder in front of me. I sat in silence as he flipped through the pages showing me different options for my father's cremation and then pointed to an illustration of an elaborate mahogany casket lined in silk. "This would be lovely along with the embroidered silk shirt," he said. "I don't think you want the simple pine box for your father." I wondered what my father needed a silk shirt for if he was being cremated. And, as Michael and I had very little money and I didn't know whether my father had anything left in his estate, I steeled myself and chose the least expensive options. The funeral director became cool and curt in his responses, and I felt guilty at my lack of outward show of emotion.

Later that morning, as I opened the door to my father's apartment with the keys salvaged from his pant pockets, I was hit with the familiar dusky smell of his aging bachelorhood. His art books, psychoanalytic literature, and prints by Brueghel, Paul Klee, and Joan Miró were all in his living room. His Go game set up on the board appeared to be in mid-game and was surrounded by open Japanese Go magazines on the wobbly round coffee table atop the red Bokhara carpet. His bathroom was almost empty, apart from a stiff shaving brush, a razor, and a nearly empty bottle of aspirin. Towels lay strewn about on the floor, stiff for lack of washing. After I looked through my father's apartment for a few minutes, Michael called out to me that someone was knocking at the door. One of my father's patients, an elegantly dressed middle-aged woman, stood expectantly at the doorstep ready for her psychoanalytic session.

When I told her in my broken German that my father had just died, she turned and ran shrieking down the spiral staircase. I pinned a note to the door announcing his death.

On his desk in a silver filigree frame stood a portrait of a young blonde woman holding a violin. I didn't recognize her and tossed the picture into the wastebasket. Also on his desk sat the ceramic box with the etched enamel Japanese landscape that I remembered from his study in Berkeley. It was empty. In one of his desk drawers I found, bundled by year in frayed twine, all the earnest childhood letters I had written since his return to Germany ten years earlier. That evening I read them all, remembering the parts of my life that I couldn't articulate in these letters, my struggles with my hearing disability and my social life. Then I threw the letters into the garbage.

In a cabinet in the living room I found several boxes stuffed with the many drafts of the book he had been working on all my life: "A Dialogue between Karl Marx and Sigmund Freud," laboriously handwritten with a fountain pen in his indecipherable shorthand. At various times over the years, he'd described this project to me: What would Marx and Freud have said to each other if they'd ever met? How would Freud have psychoanalyzed Marx? Should their dialogue be written as a play? Should it be written in English for an American audience? Clearly, after twenty years he still hadn't been able to finish their conversation. I set the boxes aside to give to an acquaintance of his who had expressed interest in them.

In another drawer, I found my father's correspondence with Albert Einstein and Bertrand Russell concerning my father's 1948 paper, "A Method to Enforce World Peace" in which he supported the establishment of a world government. He'd tried to persuade Einstein and Russell to agree with his position that Russia should be encouraged to join such a government. I thought these letters might be valuable one day, maybe Elliot and I could sell them at an auction house, so I kept them. Over the next week Michael and I efficiently sold my father's books and car, and we donated his suits, shoes, shirts, and bow ties to a local charity. Elliot and I inherited only the $12,000 left in my father's bank account; Michael and I would use our half to start our life in London.

On our last night in his apartment, the space totally empty except for the old mattress on the floor we slept on, my father appeared to me in a dream. Refreshed from a vacation, he was excited to see me and gave me his usual big bear hug.

"My dear Claudia," he murmured. Then he looked around his empty apartment and asked, horrified, "How could you dispose of me so cavalierly?" I woke up ashamed of my lack of outward emotion.

My father's death left me feeling numb. It didn't seem real and I couldn't weep. Because so many years always passed between our visits, for me, he'd gradually started to fade from my life when he left Berkeley when I was eleven. It was only years later in therapy that I could properly grieve the loss of my father and heal my disappointment over his lack of support and involvement in my life.

Chapter Twenty-One

Back in London we moved into our apartment and Michael began his master's program at the Courtauld Institute of Art. To my surprise I didn't adjust easily to our new life in England. The apartment, located between Muswell Hill and East Finchley, two suburbs in north London, sat directly over the intersection between two very busy, noisy streets. One was a major road leading to the north of England, and all day and night trucks braked to a screeching halt at the red light and then started up again with a great roar that rattled our windows.

The building had no insulation, so the apartment was cold and damp. Coal, which we needed to light our kitchen and living room fireplaces, was scarce and expensive due to the ongoing miners' strike and to bring it into the apartment meant clambering down three flights of stairs to the basement and then back up lugging the coal in buckets. The coal fire sent dust throughout the apartment and created a gray film that covered every surface. At night, a sodium vapor streetlight outside our bedroom window cast a surreal amber glow into the room, and that only further darkened my mood. Because I couldn't use the phone, I had to rely on Michael to answer and make calls on my behalf, and I hated feeling dependent. Adding to my frustration, it took over an hour and a half to get from our apartment to anywhere in central London; first the twenty-minute walk to the tube station, then the ride on the old Northern subway line closer to the center of town, and finally a change or two of trains or buses to our destination.

I tried to gain traction in my life in London and started by taking a job at the local branch of a Lloyd's bank where I typed up foreign exchange transactions. My piano playing fingers were fast, and I didn't need to hear to do the job, but it was very repetitive and boring. In my spare time, I threw myself into sewing curtains for the rooms in our apartment and made an elaborate brocade bedspread, complete with corded piping. Hoping to meet people, I took classes in calligraphy and urban photography. I set up a darkroom in the kitchen with equipment I'd brought with me from Berkeley and went out on photo shoots in central London with a new friend from one of my classes.

Meanwhile Michael was blissfully immersed in his program, and he enthusiastically shared with me what he was learning about medieval architecture. We went on several weekend excursions to study the Romanesque and Gothic architecture of famous cathedrals throughout England. Because I hardly knew anyone in London, I relied on him greatly for connection and contact. But, as an introvert, he didn't seek out friends and seemed happy with just our close companionship. I desperately wished he would bring some people into our lives.

One evening, as Michael and I sat over dinner, I said, "There's a piano shop on the Archway Road. I'll go and see what kind of piano I can buy with the $1,000 my mother and John gave me."

Michael was silent, poking at his overcooked peas. Neither of us knew how to cook, so our dinners were basic affairs, often consisting of peas and hamburger meat. Then he looked up at me.

"Actually, you have $500 for a piano."

"But they gave me $1,000."

"We're married now, so we should split all our money. I already used $500 to buy art history books."

"But they gave *me* $1,000 to get a piano. It wasn't meant for books. Can't you go to the Courtauld library for books?"

"All our money is now community property, so I get half of the $1,000, and I can use it however I want. And I want art history books."

Stunned, I didn't argue further. Maybe he was right, but I didn't want to acknowledge the devastation I felt at his lack of generosity, and I tried to put the matter out of my mind.

While continuing my temporary job at the bank, I applied to the master's program at the Institute of Archaeology and to the photography program at the Royal Academy of Art. As I waited for the results, I took time off from the bank and volunteered at two archaeological digs of Roman remains in the cathedral towns of York and Lincoln.

While I enjoyed excavating and photographing Roman mosaics and learning about the Roman occupation of Britain two thousand years earlier, as usual I had trouble socializing in the noisy dining rooms and on the sites where everyone was spread out working in individual trenches. I couldn't understand the volunteers who shouted out their discoveries or their jokes and stories. Having no friends, I felt isolated and lonely, and I missed Michael's warm camaraderie. It reminded me of my experience at the camp in Germany, and I thought again about whether there was a connection between depression and social isolation caused by hearing loss. I considered looking into new hearing aids; there must be some new advancements by now. But the hearing aids that would work with a severe hearing loss cost thousands of dollars for a pair and weren't covered by insurance, so I gave up on that idea for the time being.

My mood brightened when I returned to London to find letters informing me that I'd been accepted into both graduate programs. I was interested in photography, and I thought that program, which would allow me to rely on my visual skills rather than on being able to hear, might be a better choice than the archaeology program. But the photography program was three years long and, I discovered, was going to cost a lot of money for fees and photographic equipment. We didn't have the money, so with some misgivings, I opted for the one-year program at the Institute of Archaeology.

Adding to my extreme loneliness, Michael shut down sexually shortly after we arrived in London. He no longer initiated lovemaking and was irritated and nonresponsive when I did. Before I knew it, six months had passed since he'd last touched me. I tried to talk to him about it, but he completely refused to discuss the issue. This shutdown was very painful and foreign territory for me—so different from how things had been between us for the two and a half years in Berkeley. I didn't understand what it was about returning to England that would result in such a change in him. I suggested we see a therapist, but to my dismay he adamantly refused.

One gray afternoon we went for a picnic on Hampstead Heath overlooking central London. As we lay on the damp grass, I tentatively tried once again.

"What's going on? Why don't you want to have sex anymore? Is it me?"

He stared off into the distance and then said quietly, "I like men." I was stunned. In Berkeley he'd told me of a brief fling he had with Robert, his physical education teacher—but I'd dismissed it as standard fare among British schoolboys.

"Have you been with other men?" I put down my sandwich, having completely lost my appetite.

"Yes, but not since I met you." He rolled over and looked at me intently.

"When did this start?"

"When I was fourteen Robert seduced me once when we were alone in the locker room, but I really liked it, so it continued on and off for three years. Then I had a number of relationships with men while I was at Oxford." This news shattered me. I really didn't want to hear more, but I needed to know more.

"Were you with women too?"

"Yes."

"Why didn't you tell me all this before we got married?" A wave of anger rippled through my body.

Michael paused and looked away. "I wanted to tell you during the est training, but I was afraid I'd lose you. I thought I could just erase this part of my life and not let it affect our relationship."

"Is this why you can't have sex with me?"

"Yes." He hesitated. "I miss sex with men. It's different than with you. I thought that by marrying you, I could make my desire for men go away, but since we got back to England my attraction to men has returned. I don't think I can change this."

The wind picked up and turned icy cold. He reached for my hand and went on, "What would you think about having an open relationship? I'd see men, but you wouldn't have to know about it unless you wanted to."

I was sick with pain. I wasn't sure whether to cry or get angry. "No, I can't be with you while you're having sex with men," I insisted. "That's not the kind of marriage I want." This was new territory for me. It was the mid-1970s and I hardly knew anyone else who was gay.

He looked miserably down at his sandwich. It began to drizzle. We packed up the remains of our picnic, neatly folded our blanket, and stood up to leave.

"We need to see a therapist," I said. I was holding on to a last shred of hope.

He turned his back to me and started to walk ahead. "If you want to see a therapist to sort out your feelings, that's fine. But I know how I feel, and I don't need to see a therapist."

I was angry. "So, you're saying it is up to me to accept this situation if we're to remain married?"

"Yes."

It was all moving so fast. His adamant refusal to see a therapist with me turned my heart into lead. I knew then that my marriage was over.

The next few months were surreal as it became clear that Michael wasn't going to talk further about our relationship. He was warm and affectionate and continued to share all that he was learning in his art history program, and we regularly attended concerts, films, and art exhibits. But he continued to show no interest in sex. We pretended that everything was normal between us, but I was quietly biding my time until I was emotionally ready to leave him. I busied myself as much as possible with my archaeology classes.

Because coal was so expensive, the Institute of Archaeology was barely heated, so during the late fall and winter months, even indoors everyone was dressed in overcoats, hats, and gloves. The cold just added to my despondent mood, and to add to my misery, I found I had a harder time hearing at the Institute of Archaeology than I had in lectures at UC Berkeley. The roar of the double decker buses outside on the busy street often drowned out whoever was speaking during discussions. Fortunately, some of the classes were in the form of private tutorials with a professor and just one other student. I made some friends and did well in the program, but I was thoroughly miserable. I felt I was living a lie, acting normally with Michael and my few friends at the Institute while at the same time secretly planning my escape from England.

One snowy Saturday in February I accompanied Michael to the bus stop. He was off to attend an art history conference for the weekend at Oxford. From the back of the bus, he cheerily waved goodbye to me out the window. I smiled and returned his wave, but I knew it would probably be the last time I saw him. With a fractured heart, I dashed back to the apartment and got to work. I booked a one-way flight to San Francisco and sent a few packages of clothes and books to Berkeley. I stuffed various mementoes, photographs, and my camera equipment into two suitcases, locked the exterior door to our apartment, and dropped the key with a note through the mailbox slot. *By the time you read this note, I'll be halfway across the Atlantic,* I wrote. I felt badly about leaving without telling him but knew it was the only way I could move on. I spent my last night in London with a friend from the Institute of Archaeology. Tossing and turning on her sofa, I tried to distract my thoughts from Michael, worrying instead about whether my suitcases were too heavy and if I'd have to pay a hefty fine.

The next morning at the airport check-in counter, I stood behind an American businessman dressed in an elegant gray suit holding a light carry-on bag.

"How're you?" he asked, picking up on my anxiety.

"I've just left my husband, and I think I'm way over the weight limit," I burst out, pointing to my bulging suitcases.

"Here, let me take one of those; I'll check it as mine. That way you won't risk an excess luggage fee."

He then led me into the Business Class VIP room, ordered me a gin and tonic, and left me alone. I felt calmer and was profoundly grateful to him; his kindness gave me hope for the future. Once on the plane I gazed out the window at the fog below while *Jaws*, a welcome distraction, was playing on the TV monitors above the aisles. Then, halfway across the Atlantic, the clouds parted to reveal an impossibly deep cobalt blue sky. At the sight of nature's miraculous beauty, my heart soared. I had grieved my extreme loneliness and difficult relationship with Michael the entire three years in England, but now I was ready to begin to put this painful time behind me and look towards the future. As I stared out the window at the vast expanse of sky, I realized that what made it possible to leave Michael was that I was finally able to forgive myself for having made the mistake of marrying him. I'd done it against my better judgment, and I vowed that I would trust myself more, that I wouldn't go against my intuition again.

I knew I would go through a painful adjustment when I returned to Berkeley, that I'd miss Michael's warmth and supportiveness of me, our closeness and all the interests we shared. But for the first time in a long while I was optimistic about what lay ahead; I was ready to heal and begin again.

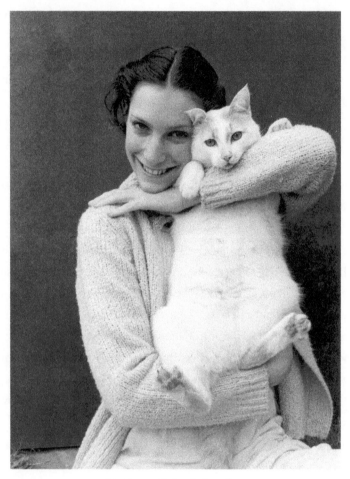

Monica with her beloved cat

Chapter Twenty-Two

I embraced my mother, John, and Monica with relieved bear hugs at the airport. After three years away I was thrilled to lay eyes on Monica, who was now eleven years old. On the car ride home she couldn't stop hugging me and holding my hand. I wanted to live near my family, partly so I could renew my connection with my little sister. A friend found me a tiny one-room apartment in Oakland and helped me secure a job as a typist and receptionist in a medium-sized law firm. I was overjoyed I was so quickly landing on my feet and that I was able to live in my beloved East Bay Area.

But right away my new job proved to be painfully challenging. I was barely able to hear on the phone even with the telecoil on my hearing aids, not an ideal job for someone with a severe hearing loss who relied heavily on lipreading. In my job interview I hadn't told my prospective boss about my disability as I knew I'd be unlikely to get the job, which I desperately needed. In the future, businesses would be set up with technical and other kinds of accommodations for people with disabilities, but at this point the installation of simple volume adapters for office phones was still years away. I did the best I could with the limited amount I was able to hear, but with a sense of shame I knew I was not very effective at my job.

I quickly became friends with the other secretaries in the firm, eating all my lunches with them. This gave me a welcome sense of belonging.

"Where're you from?" one of them asked. "You have an accent. Are you French or Swedish?"

People had often asked me what my accent was, not always picking up that I had a speech defect from my hearing loss. As I couldn't hear the sibilant sounds, the "s's," the "sch's," "ch's," etc., I didn't articulate them as well. I was also told that I vocalized more from the back of my throat rather than projecting from the front. I began to use this question of my accent as an opportunity to tell people about my hearing loss. But in this case, I didn't explain because I didn't want to jeopardize my job.

"I lived in England the last three years, maybe that's it," I answered.

When Angela, one of the older secretaries, learned I'd just left my husband and was figuring out how to get a divorce, she took me under her wing and offered to help me file the paperwork. Practically all the secretaries in the firm had done their own divorces without the use of attorneys, and their help meant my divorce wouldn't cost much. Angela told me which civil code box to tick off on the form as grounds for the divorce, and I sent the paperwork to Michael to sign. A few weeks later I received a letter from him.

There's a problem with the paperwork you sent, he wrote. *I know we had our difficulties, but "incurable insanity" was not one of them!*

I had to laugh. I guessed that he, too, was amused. I had apparently checked the wrong civil code box, so I filed the paperwork again, this time checking the box for "irreconcilable differences," and, in six months our divorce was finalized.

I heard from a mutual friend that Michael was lonely and depressed, and I felt sad for him. Although I missed him greatly, I'd done most of the hard grieving while we were still together. I was over my anger about him concealing from me that he was gay; mostly I was relieved to have that very painful period of my life behind me.

My master's in British archaeology was useless in the Bay Area, so I was highly motivated to go to graduate school to gain some practical skills to help me land a good job. Since my return, Elliot and I immediately reconnected, catching up with each other's lives over long conversations. He was attending the two-year master's program at the Graduate School of Public Policy at UC Berkeley and encouraged me to check it out. I hardly knew what public policy was, and I certainly didn't have the background in statistics or economics that would have been helpful in the program. Nevertheless, I mustered my courage and walked over to the school's office for an informal interview with one of their professors. Two years later, at age twenty-seven, I graduated with a master's in public policy and took a job at Pacific Gas and Electric (PG&E) in their energy conservation department.

I was part of a group that designed market research surveys to evaluate PG&E's programs encouraging customers to reduce their energy consumption. This was the late '70s, and energy conservation was all the rage. Although my heart wasn't in the quantitative aspects of the work, I was grateful to have a steady job and the independence that came with being able to support myself. The meetings at the conservation unit were formal with little crosstalk, so I was able to follow and contribute to the discussions. And because much of my work required writing interoffice memos in my cubicle, I was largely able to avoid using the phone. I did well at my job and managed to hide my hearing loss from my boss and teammates. I was afraid it might jeopardize my job if they knew.

I became great friends with my teammates in the conservation unit, eating lunch with them every day and going for hikes and parties on the weekends. I told my friends outside of my job about my hearing loss, which was in keeping with my practice over the past few years of being more honest about my disability. I was now fully settled back in my northern California life, and my heart swelled with a welcome sense of connection and belonging.

I rented a charming, woodsy mother-in-law cottage in Berkeley, and a family friend loaned me her Steinway grand piano, which I squeezed

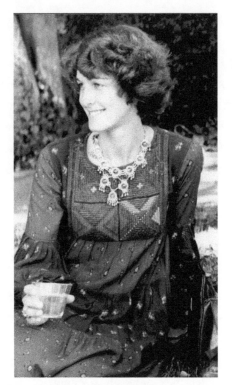

Home from England;
photo credit: Donna May

into the cottage's little sitting area next to the kitchen. I started taking lessons again, and when I came home from work, as dusk turned into night, I dove into practicing Beethoven's late piano sonatas. My teacher, Julian White, a well-known Bay Area pianist, hosted informal recitals at his house in the Berkeley Hills where we students performed for each other. For the first time in my life, I had an abundance of friends—from graduate school, my job, a women's group I'd joined two years earlier, and my piano group. I was happy.

Then my life, at age twenty-nine, took another big turn. I met Sam. PG&E paid for those of us who held jobs involving technical writing to attend a writing class at UC Berkeley, and Sam and I were sent to the same workshop. At that time, I was in an ethnic clothing phase and showed up at the first class dressed in a long navy blue pleated skirt with brown boots, a white Guatemalan blouse with red embroidery, and a navy-blue French beret. I caught Sam gazing at me, and I was attracted to his open and friendly face. He had brown hair, gray eyes, and a large nose that I later learned he inherited from his Palestinian father. A few days later when he phoned to ask me out, I had an intuitive flash: *I'm going to marry this man.* He was an economist, rising quickly through the ranks in PG&E's rate department, and he told me that he was planning to leave PG&E soon to start his own energy conservation consulting firm.

Quickly we formed a tight bond. We shared a love of nature and went on many hikes and exploratory trips throughout northern California. Sam encouraged me to keep up with photography and we went to many art exhibits. Music wasn't in his background, but he enthusiastically learned from me as we attended concerts, and he sat and listened to me practice in the evenings after work. He was a passionate collector of Turkish kilims and Caucasian carpets and exposed me to the world of Middle Eastern textiles by taking me to rug fairs and auctions. In addition, Sam shared his love of Sufism, the mystical branch of Islam, and would read Sufi stories aloud to me as we cuddled together on the couch. I fell deeply in love with him.

He was very different from Michael—ambitious, three years younger than I, and from a blue-collar family in Chicago. His father had lost family land and orange orchards when the State of Israel was created and his family sought refuge in Jordan. At the end of high school, Sam's father had had the good fortune to receive a Quaker scholarship to study at Swarthmore college in the United States. Sam's mother was American but had grown up in rural China as the daughter of missionaries. She'd met Sam's father at Swarthmore, but when they became pregnant with Sam, they had to drop out of college. They moved to Chicago where his father worked a forklift during the day and studied engineering at night.

Fortunately, as neither Sam nor I had been raised with religion, our divergent backgrounds weren't a source of conflict for either of us or for our families. Sam's unique background, talents in economics and mathematics, and spiritual interests intrigued me. I was also excited about his plans to start his own consulting business because I knew he was too independent to last long term in a conventional company like PG&E. And like Michael and my past boyfriends, he took my hearing loss matter-of-factly. I could tell he felt protective. He often turned to me to explain what had just been said in a social situation, and he listened sympathetically to reports of my struggles with the phone and meetings at work. As in the past, starting with Elliot, then friends, and later Michael, I had a much-needed ally who acted as an important interface between me and the world, explaining what was going on around me and sometimes making phone calls on my behalf. Soon Sam moved into my cottage, and we started sharing expenses, with him generously paying for things I couldn't afford.

After two years at PG&E, I took a job at the Council of State Governments in San Francisco where I was part of a team supporting Western state governments on regional policy issues, such as State and Native American water rights, public lands, highway transportation, and prison reform. I found the work much more interesting than at PG&E, and I quickly became friends with the other employees. My hearing loss made parts of my job challenging, and again, I didn't explicitly tell my boss or teammates about my disability.

Our staff of six professionals was responsible for organizing and hosting conferences several times a year throughout the West for Western state governors, legislators, attorneys general, and legislative analysts. Part of my task was to help conduct meetings of thirty or so legislators, write summary memos, and draft resolutions that they would vote on the following day. At these meetings I struggled

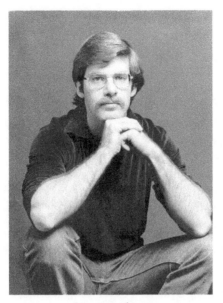

Sam, age thirty

to follow the legislators' rapid-paced, free-wheeling discussions and wisecracks to extract what was important to include in my memos, but I became skilled in surreptitiously gleaning from other staff members what had been said.

One afternoon at a conference in Jackson Hole after a heated meeting on gasoline taxation, I sidled over to Curt, one of the legislators' staff also in attendance, and asked, as nonchalantly as possible, "What'd you think of that discussion?" I desperately hoped I would get a recap of what had just taken place. *Were the legislators inclined to agree or disagree about the proposal under consideration?* I wondered.

"Well, they seemed pretty energized, more than usual, I'd say. We'll see what they decide in tomorrow's vote," he answered.

But I needed to figure out from him, *now*, how most of the legislators were leaning on the issue and what the pros and cons were to write my memo for them to review in the morning.

"Shall we go downstairs to the café for a bite to eat?" I asked.

As the coffee and bread were placed in front of us, I asked Curt, "What's your opinion, what do you think they'll decide on tomorrow?"

To my great relief, he finally opened up, and, over the background noise of the café, I strained to hear as best I could what he had to say about the meeting. The legislators seemed to be equally divided about the proposal, so I'd have to argue the advantages and disadvantages of both sides in my draft. For now, I had the information I needed. But I always felt I was precariously skating on thin ice being so dependent on the unwitting willingness of others to give me information while at the same time trying desperately to hide my periodic cluelessness.

Back in the office, most of the work entailed researching and writing reports. This was less stressful than the conferences we hosted, but I had to make frequent phone calls. As in graduate school, I was often tense before making a call for I never knew whether I'd be able to hear and obtain the information I needed to do my work. I continued, as much as possible, to keep my invisible disability a secret at work. At this time, invisible disabilities in the workplace were simply not discussed.

One evening over dinner after a particularly frustrating day, I confided in Sam the extent of my struggles with the phone and the meetings.

"Why don't you go and check out what new technology there might be in hearing aids," Sam said. "It's been eight years since you got new ones, right? Hearing aids are bound to be better by now."

"I don't think anything has changed since the last pair I got before I moved to England," I answered.

Despite my protests, his suggestion made me excited about the possibility of some new improvements. But I also steeled myself against possible disappointment. Not much had noticeably changed for me in the hearing aids I'd gotten since my first behind-the-ear hearing aids when I was eleven, which had been a huge improvement from the hearing aids of my early childhood. Also, high-end hearing aids were very expensive and not covered by health insurance.

"But what about the cost?" I asked.

"Don't worry about the cost," Sam said. "We'll figure out a way to pay for them."

Sam and his easygoing support made me feel extremely lucky. I knew there were so many people who simply couldn't afford the latest hearing aids.

Besides new hearing aids, I needed new acrylic ear molds as the ones I had been wearing for years now had shrunk and were quite loose. My hearing loss was severe enough that discreet in-the-ear canal aids weren't effective. And the new open canal molds that allowed more air into the ear also didn't work. I needed, essentially, customized plugs to contain the amplified sound within my ear.

With the molds I'd been wearing for years, whenever my ears wriggled because I was chewing food or smiling, I'd hear the awful high-pitched feedback whistle. The molds had to fit tightly enough to prevent the whistle, but if they were too tight, my ears broke out in painful blisters and calluses. There was a sweet spot between too loose and too tight, and from a lifetime of experience, I knew this sweet spot wasn't easy to find. But, although I dreaded adjusting to new hearing aids and molds, it was time.

I had a hearing test with a new audiologist and when he saw the results, he said, "I'm amazed that you do so well at your job, despite your level of hearing loss." We were both hopeful that new hearing aids would be an improvement, and we were excited the day I tried them on. But once again, I was disappointed; I didn't hear better than before. The audiologist tinkered with some adjustments, but it was still as hard as ever to distinguish speech in a noisy background. In addition, although the telecoil boosting the magnetic signal from the landline phones was now stronger, so was the buzz that came through the hearing aids, making it difficult to hear the speaker at the other end of the line.

In my free time, I happily busied myself taking piano lessons, spending time with friends, and going on weekend hikes with Sam. I also started attending photography classes at night. I loved photography, and I wanted to make up for having declined for financial reasons the photography program at the Royal Academy in London. I gravitated towards portrait photography as I had spent a lifetime of looking at and reading faces.

I enrolled in a class on studio portrait lighting taught by G. Paul Bishop, a well-known Bay Area portrait photographer in his seventies who created exquisite black and white portraits. He was skilled at revealing a subject's character through his sensitive portrayal of their expression. As well as portraits of the general public, he was known for his luminous photographs of some of UC Berkeley's Nobel laureates and of various famous poets and artists. When I first walked in the door of his small home studio and saw his portraits displayed on the walls, I knew I wanted to make portraits like his. Paul was retiring and not taking on new students, but over the next few weeks I persistently appealed to him.

"I just love your work, and I want to learn directly from you!" I gushed one afternoon after class.

"No, really, I can't take on a new student," he said.

"Maybe just a few lessons? I'd work really hard."

"Sorry. Good night."

I tried a few more times over the next several weeks. "Your portraiture really moves me. I want to be able to take pictures like yours. Can you make an exception for me? I really want to study with you."

"Well, you're doing excellent work in class," he said finally. "Do you have a darkroom?"

"I'm in the process of setting one up, but I'd really like your help. I want to buy an enlarger, and I need your suggestions as to what kind I should buy." I saw that my shameless appeals for his help was finally melting his resistance.

"Well, OK. We should probably start by reviewing how you

develop your film. And then we should go out and get you a good enlarger with a proper lens. Would you be ready to start next week?"

I was thrilled. I ended up studying with Paul weekly for the next two years, and he became a cherished mentor and friend. With his help, I bought what I needed to set up a darkroom in the laundry room of the cottage, and I spent many happy hours under the orange safelight developing and printing negatives from photo shoots in his studio. Once a week, we worked companionably together in his tiny kitchen darkroom experimenting with different developer chemicals and papers in search of the combination that would yield the best black and white print possible.

One evening I showed Paul some black and white prints I'd made from photographs I had taken of two girls playing dress up. One girl looked directly at the camera, and the other looked off to the side revealing an elegant profile. The photograph was arresting, and my heart swelled with love and pride for what I had made. *Yes! These are good!* I thought. In addition to the composition being strong, the prints had fine photographic detail across the entire black and white tonal range, and I knew Paul would be pleased.

"What do you think of these?" I asked, spreading them out on the coffee table in front him.

"Oh, these are delightful," he gushed. "They positively sing!" His comment filled me with joy. *I am becoming a very good photographer,* I thought.

When I was thirty, after Sam and I had lived together for a year in the little cottage, we bought a house using money Sam had saved. It was brown shingled with a Mediterranean style interior in the Berkeley Hills under a stand of redwood trees at the edge of Tilden Park. After two wonderful years playing the lovely Steinway grand, I'd had to return it, but after the loan financing for the house was concluded, we had some money left over that we hadn't expected. Sam surprised me by saying, "Go get yourself a good piano." *So different from Michael,* I thought. With our new house, garden, piano, Sam's textiles decorating the interiors, and new friends, I was on top of the world with my new life.

Sam started growing his energy conservation consulting business, and I continued working at the Council of State Governments, traveling throughout the Western states to conferences, doing the best I could at the meetings. We knocked down the wall between the two small bedrooms in the back of our house to convert the space into a portrait studio, and once again I set up my darkroom in the laundry room. Paul Bishop referred some clients to me, and I started taking black and white portraits of children, individuals, and families during my spare time. I loved doing portraits and I was thrilled to earn some extra money through my own creative work.

Because photography is so visual, it turned out to be a wonderful art form for me. But one part of photography proved challenging. During portrait sessions, when I looked down at the camera to change film or alter the camera's settings, I couldn't keep up an easy banter with clients because I couldn't lipread and change film at the same time. I improvised a solution by doing most of the talking myself. That way I wouldn't have to strain to hear my clients while taking pictures.

When I was thirty-two, Sam and I got married in our back garden under our large loquat tree, surrounded by our friends and relatives. Paul Bishop's son, a friend and also a fine photographer, shot our wedding photos, and my piano teacher played my favorite Beethoven bagatelle for the ceremony. For our honeymoon, we trekked for three weeks around the Annapurna mountain range in Nepal, climbing over a pass of almost eighteen thousand feet. In the seven years since I'd left Michael in London, my life had changed in ways I couldn't have imagined.

And there was still more good news. One evening a year later, I skipped over to Sam, who was working at his desk, and held up the strip from the pregnancy test I had just taken. I was pregnant! Sam stood up and threw his arms around me. During a celebratory dinner in downtown Berkeley, we discussed how we'd handle a baby while I was working in San Francisco and traveling.

"Why don't you quit your job and just focus on photography?" Sam said. "You could work from home."

In that moment, a lifetime burden of compensating for and often hiding my hearing loss lifted from my shoulders. *Photography and taking care of a baby, that I can do,* I thought with a profound relief. But I did have one worry.

"How will I hear our baby cry at night?" I asked Sam. "You know I don't hear a thing without my hearing aids."

"I'll hear the baby. And I can do some of the feedings too," Sam said.

The next many years were profoundly fulfilling. Sam and I cherished parenting our daughter, Mira, and we made friends with other couples with young children, some of whom also became photography clients. I continued to show my work to Paul Bishop, and soon my portrait photography business was thriving. I scheduled photo shoots in the room we had remodeled in the back of the house and did my darkroom work in our laundry room. This made it possible for me to work around Mira's naps, and later, around her part-time day care.

By the time Mira was three years old, I'd outgrown our home studio, and I rented a studio space in West Berkeley. Now that I wasn't dependent on an employer for a job, I felt freer to tell people I was hard of hearing, including my clients who would now understand why I wasn't always able to converse with them when they posed across the room from me or gathered in large groupings for family portraits.

But I was by no means free from the challenges resulting from not being able to hear well. One bittersweet incident took place one morning when Mira was six. I was driving her and her friend Sarah to their Waldorf school when Mira piped up from the backseat.

"Mommy, we wanna know, what's God?" she asked.

As I turned left onto busy San Pablo Avenue in Oakland, I thought, *Oh wow, this is a serious question, how am I going to answer this?*

"Well, that's a very important question and there's no easy answer," I told the girls. "Some people believe he's an old man with a white beard floating in the sky, but most people don't believe that, and Daddy and I don't believe that."

Before I could go on, Mira asked, "Yeah, but what's God?" She emphasized the word "God."

"Different religions have different ideas about God. And some people believe that God doesn't exist at all. When you're older you'll have to decide for yourself what God is."

I went on for some time in this vein, giving them a cross-cultural discourse on religion and feeling rather pleased with myself. I straightened up so I could see the girls in the rearview mirror. They were both rolling their eyes, and I could see them breathing heavy, world-weary sighs.

"Yeah, yeah, we know all that stuff, but what's *God*?!"

Finally, I realized I wasn't hearing her question correctly. I pulled over into a red zone, stopped the car, and turned around to look directly at Mira.

"Sweetie, what are you asking me?"

"We want to know what 'gauze' is. Yesterday Lili went to the dentist and he put 'gauze' in her mouth!" Mira looked a bit frightened.

At last able to read her lips and distinguish between the "d" of God, from the "z" of gauze, I understood what she was saying. I turned back and lay my head down on the steering wheel and erupted into hysterical laughter. It reminded me of so many painful mis-hearings during my life, but this one was delightfully light-hearted. I pulled back onto the road and inched my way into the traffic. Despite it all, life was so very good.

Epilogue

The past thirty years have brought profoundly positive changes into my life. Being married to my generous, understanding husband Sam, and helping to raise our daughter to become a thriving young woman, have been the two most satisfying and rewarding undertakings of my life. I have a small family, but I love everyone in it. I've also cultivated a wide circle of friends, and with them I experience the kind of wonderful contact and connection I struggled with while growing up. Through my meditation practice I've learned to take pleasure in the many precious beauties of everyday life—the changing seasons, bouquets of flowers, the luminous sunsets from our window, literature, Beethoven's music.

I also have a rich creative life. In 2001, after fifteen years as a black and white fine-art portrait photographer, I earned an MFA in painting from John F. Kennedy University. Since then, I've been a professional abstract painter, incorporating oils, encaustic (a melted beeswax process), and my photographs into my work. I've created a way to combine my interests in archaeology and photography through the application of multiple layers and the buildup of history through paint and wax into my paintings, and my work is represented by an art gallery in the San Francisco Bay Area. After a long hiatus while at art school, I started playing the piano again with a close friend focusing on repertoire written for four hands. We've given several informal recitals at my home, and that's been very gratifying. All these elements have added up to a very rich life, one I'm grateful for beyond measure.

As happily focused as I am on the present and future, I do spend some time thinking of everything I went through because of my hearing challenges. So much of life really comes down to timing, to luck. If I'd been born twenty or thirty years earlier, I would have struggled with even more rudimentary hearing aids than those I used during my early childhood, which were cumbersome and awkward. But I know how fortunate I was that they were as good as they were. That said, if I'd been born at a different time, my mother might not have been prescribed a toxic medication and I wouldn't have experienced any hearing loss at all. And if I'd been born forty years later, I'd have benefitted from much more sophisticated technology. I would have had digital hearing aids from the beginning and would have grown up in a culture that much more widely accepts, respects, and accommodates people with disabilities. But overall, I feel I was dealt a pretty good hand.

During my lifetime, two major movements, mutually influencing each other, dramatically improved the quality of my life. The first, inspired by the Civil Rights movement from 1954 to 1968, was the disability rights movement, whose goal was equal opportunities and equal rights for all people with disabilities. The Center for Independent Living was founded in Berkeley in 1972, sparking a worldwide independent living movement that advocated for the use of supportive services like assistive technology, income supplements, and personal aid to improve opportunities for those with disabilities. I'll never forget the rush of joy I felt the first time I saw a sidewalk curb that had been transformed into ramps for wheelchair access. Seeing people in wheelchairs traveling independently increased public awareness and acceptance of disabilities.

Deafness and hearing loss have even been featured in many films over the past decades, such as the immensely popular "Children of a Lesser God," "The Piano," and more recently, "CODA" and "Sound of Metal." But it took several decades for an increased awareness of disabilities to result in the passage of the Americans with Disabilities Act (ADA) of 1990. The ADA, which includes a requirement for reasonable accommodation on job sites for people who are deaf or disabled, profoundly improved modes of communication for deaf people, including the use of telecommunication devices for the deaf (TTYs), sign language interpreters, and closed captioning. Closed captioning has made an enormous difference in my life, finally making it possible for me to understand and enjoy movies and news on TV. Being able to keep up with what my peers are watching makes me feel much more connected to the world.

The academic landscape for students with hearing loss has also dramatically improved. In 1994, Assembly Bill 1836, "The Deaf Children's Bill of Rights," was signed into law in California by then Governor Pete Wilson. This historic legislation acknowledges the essential need for children who are deaf and hard of hearing to be educated in an environment that respects and uses their preferred mode of communication. The law also emphasizes the need for hard of hearing students to be able to participate in all school programs, including afterschool social and athletic functions, and the social life of lunch and recess. I have often thought with sadness how much happier and easier my school life would have been if I had grown up in the post "Deaf Children's Bill of Rights" era.

Now, in most public schools, disabled students are supported through an Individual Education Plan (IEP) drawn up for them by a committee of specialists who work with teachers to create individualized plans and help arrange for needed accommodations. For deaf or hard of hearing students, note takers and sign language interpreters are provided as needed. Teachers wear FM devices or use other technology to transmit sound directly to students' hearing aids. All films and videos must be captioned and teachers write on projectors that enlarge images on a whiteboard in front of the class. This means a teacher is always facing the class when speaking, while at the same time students can read what the teacher has written. What a difference from what I struggled through!

Some classrooms are configured in a U shape so all the students can see each other. Teachers are encouraged to speak loudly and to repeat students' comments and questions so everyone can understand them wherever they're sitting. Teachers also discuss with students their optimal spot to sit where they can hear and lipread the best. Disabled students are allocated more time to complete assignments and tests, and students are coached and encouraged to advocate for themselves, to speak up when they don't understand something. I certainly could have used that kind of training and encouragement.

Despite these major gains, deafness is an invisible disability, and disabilities, even today, carry a stigma. Unseen disabilities—certain mental disorders, brain injuries, chronic fatigue syndrome, and diabetes, to name just a few—are often not acknowledged and discussed in the workplace, leading to marginalization and isolation by employers and peers. Interestingly, in Coqual's 2017 study, "Disabilities and Inclusion," a full 30 percent of the American professional workforce fits the federal definition of having some kind of disability, and the majority are keeping that status a secret. Only 39 percent of employees with disabilities disclose their disability to their manager. Even fewer disclose it to their teams (24 percent) and to HR (21 percent). There's still an onus about having a disability and concern about how this difference might impact the disabled person's work life. I understand this all too well. There's still progress to be made in accepting disabilities in the workforce.

The second trend that's had a profound impact on my life was the explosion in hearing technologies brought about by the digital revolution of the past twenty years. In the late 1990s, I obtained my first all-digital hearing aids, and they made it easier for me to hear in noisy situations, always the most challenging situation for those with hearing loss. With digital hearing aids it's possible to adjust the level of amplification to selected frequencies. For most people with hearing loss, there needs to be a greater boost of amplification in the higher frequencies where speech resides. In addition, digital aids can be programmed with several different frequency profiles to be used in various hearing situations, such as a noisy restaurant, a concert hall, and a quiet gathering. Just recently I purchased new powerful hearing aids which have been set up with three different programs: one for "normal" or quiet situations, one for music—which I love because it brings out more of the bass frequencies—and one that I use in very noisy situations. Everyone's brain processes sound differently, and I've had to patiently go through a process of trial and error as my audiologist adjusts my new hearing aids in search of the optimal setup for me.

But the recent development I find most exciting is the ability to connect hearing aids via Bluetooth and various assistive listening devices to smart phones, computers, and TVs, so the sound is transmitted directly to hearing aids. My new hearing aids have these new connectivity features. For the first time ever, I'm now able to have clear and stress-free phone conversations via Bluetooth through my iPhone. I am so thankful for this innovation, but I also think back with some sadness at my many years of struggles with the phone when I was an adolescent and in my early professional life.

Another recent technological advance that has directly bene-fitted me has been the development of Assistive Listening Devices (ALDs)—FM radio, Infrared, Bluetooth, or other wireless devices that help people hear in noisy situations and classroom settings. Now I sometimes hang a wireless device around Sam's or a friend's neck to better hear in a restaurant that isn't too noisy. This small three-inch disc wirelessly transmits their voice from the device's microphone below their mouth directly into receivers built into my hearing aids. If the background noise is not too intense, the speaker's voice comes through intelligibly above the ambient clamor. Then I can calmly lean back and relax and let the sound wash directly into my hearing aids rather than leaning forward and straining to hear. This device lifts a veil between me and the other person, allowing me to feel more connected to the world. Recently at a Thanksgiving dinner with ten people, I placed the device in the center of the table and it transmitted the group conversation directly into my hearing aids. I almost cried over the improved connection I felt to my family.

The Internet, personal computers, smart phones, and videoconferencing programs like Zoom—all byproducts of the digital revolution—have also been a huge boon for deaf and hard of hearing people, who can now sign and lipread on Zoom and similar platforms. Even with the new Bluetooth feature, I hardly use the phone these days, finding it much easier to text, email, or use Zoom. Smart phones even transcribe voice messages so I can read the gist of a message rather than struggling helplessly to make out the voice recording. In addition, there are now captioned telephones, a service whereby a hard of hearing or deaf person can talk on the phone with captioning support, as well as other speech recognition and captioning applications.

Although developed earlier, another major technological advance has been the increased use, by the late 1990s, of cochlear implants for many children and adults with profound hearing loss. The implant is a surgical procedure that installs a coil in the cochlea which stimulates the cochlear nerve. Signals are then sent to the sound processor that is worn behind the ear. This innovation has not directly affected me, however. Because I have enough residual hearing and function well enough with hearing aids and lipreading, I was never considered a candidate for the implants, but for many people with profound hearing loss, it has been extremely helpful.

Interestingly, these improvements in hearing technology have coincided with the age-related hearing loss that baby boomers are experiencing. Many adults with mild or moderate hearing loss are now able to purchase hearing aids over the counter at greatly reduced prices, making hearing aids available to people who previously couldn't afford the high cost. These hearing aids can be adjusted by the user through apps on iPhones, giving the wearer greater control over different sound profiles. This increased use of hearing aids is helping to normalize hearing loss.

Finally, there are now state-mandated programs throughout the country to screen newborns to detect hearing loss early. Thanks to these developments, infants identified to have hearing loss can be fitted with hearing aids when they're as young as six weeks old. This early intervention is vital as it can prevent nerve atrophy, and in many cases, jumpstart infants and toddlers on language development.

Because of the increased awareness and acceptance of disabilities, I'm no longer reticent about telling people about my hearing loss. It helps to explain why I don't always respond quickly or appropriately, especially when someone strikes up a conversation from behind me or in noisy situations. Letting people know I am hard of hearing means they're less likely to view me as reserved, aloof, or spaced out. And although I sometimes continue to "fake laugh" in social situations when someone makes a joke because I think it's not worth interrupting the flow to ask for the punchline to be repeated, I do it less often. These days, I'm more willing to be authentic and admit I didn't catch it. At other times I simply let the joke or comment roll off my shoulders. Passing as normal is no longer as important to me as it was when I was younger and wanted to be like everyone else—and later when I needed a job. When I do tell people about my disability, I find them sympathetic, although I know that most don't understand the myriad ways severe hearing loss impacts a life.

But even today, at times I feel a kind of invisibility. I find my friends and others forget that I have a hearing loss and will assume I can hear well in situations, such as group gatherings, when I can't. And when I take art workshops, for example, it is difficult to participate in the free-flowing, back-and-forth banter with others in the painting classes. The radio blares, people chatter away with their neighbors while painting, and I simply can't participate. I have to look away from my painting to figure out who is speaking and then try to lipread them. By then the conversation would have moved on to another person, and I wouldn't know who. It simply isn't possible for me to paint and be part of the camaraderie of the group at the same time. Mostly I just give up and work in an invisible silence.

While I've mostly become accustomed to not catching much of what is said in social situations, there are still times when I feel the minor stings of being out of the loop. Socializing in noisy restaurants continues to be very difficult. I can't enjoy the theater without reading the script ahead of time, which isn't always possible with very contemporary plays. The ALD headsets provided in some theaters are designed more for those with age-related hearing loss and so the amplification is not sufficient for me to hear. When I am with a group of friends and someone, whose face is turned away from me, makes a joke and everyone erupts in laughter, I am left out of the loop. If the person next to me turns away to make a comment, I won't grasp what they said, and it can take me awhile to catch up with the conversation. This happens regularly.

Friends sometimes tell me that when we first met, they thought I was a bit aloof or formal as I didn't respond to everything they said. That's painful to hear because I'm actually quite outgoing. I gravitate towards one-on-one interactions because they're so much easier, but I'd love to be at ease in large group conversations. Friends also tell me they forget I have a serious hearing loss because I compensate so well with lipreading. But when they forget to face me and ask a question behind my back or in a noisy group and I don't respond, they're reminded I can't hear them. It isn't a coincidence I ended up becoming an artist; most of the time I work by myself without having to rely on hearing others. I've compensated for my hearing limitations by developing an acute visual sense that has served me well as a photographer and painter.

There are many situations in which I can't have any conversation at all with people. This is often a source of distress. I can't interact with my hairdresser because I have to take out my hearing aids as she washes and cuts my hair. Same with getting a massage or being with others in a swimming pool, sauna, or hot tub. When I'm at the doctor or dentist and the staff is wearing hygienic masks, I can't lipread. And when COVID-19 swept the world, the ubiquitous mask wearing made communication profoundly frustrating; it is so painful to be unable to converse freely and connect because I can't lipread. At such times I feel thrown back to my early hearing struggles. Most of the time I accept these small but repeated frustrations and humiliations, but sometimes I feel grief at not being able to participate in the social world more fully.

Despite these difficulties I feel extremely grateful. I've largely made peace with my hearing loss. I so appreciate the life I have forged for myself, the creative endeavors I have undertaken, the adventurous travel abroad, and the many deep friendships and connections I have nurtured over the years. And now I've even written a book. I've found a path to a rich, fulfilling life.

When I was younger, the absence of sound and my efforts to understand what people said engendered loss, pain, frustration, exclusion, embarrassment, and even dishonesty. But due to technology and social advancements, and thanks in part to support from others, I learned to cope with and even take charge of my disability. I learned to stand and speak up, to reach out, to risk, to venture, to love and to forgive. I've found my place in the world. And thereby learned that acceptance is one of the sweetest sounds.

Notes

Chapter One

1. Sensorineural, or nerve-related hearing loss, refers to damage either to the tiny hair cells in the inner ear or to the nerve pathways that carry sound signals from the inner ear to the brain. This type of loss is unlike the less common conductive hearing loss due to problems with the actual structure of the ear canal or the eardrum. Some of the most common causes of sensorineural nerve damage are a side effect of certain strong antibiotics, other ototoxic medications, such as what my mother took when pregnant with me, viruses, and Meniere's disease. In older people this type of hearing loss is found to be caused by a lifetime of overexposure to loud sound.

2. If the lowest decibel range at which a person can hear sound falls between 26 and 40 decibels (dB), their hearing loss is considered mild. If a person's lowest perceptible sounds fall between 41 and 55dB, the hearing loss is moderate. Between 56 and 70 is moderate to severe, and between 71 and 90 is considered severe. And if someone can hear only sounds louder than 90 dB, their hearing loss is profound. Hearing loss tends to be greater in the higher frequencies. Unfortunately, as speech falls within the mid to high frequency range, even a person with mild or moderate overall hearing loss can have trouble comprehending speech.

3. It was important for me to be fitted with a hearing aid right away to stimulate my remaining ear fibers with sound. This would put the

nerves to work, preventing them from irreversibly atrophying further through lack of use. Because I was already four years old when I got my first hearing aid, my auditory nerves had probably already irreversibly atrophied to some extent. For this reason, the audiologist recommended wearing a custom-made mold made for each ear and alternating ears every six weeks to give each ear some experience with hearing. The hearing aid, as big as a deck of cards, would clip onto my undershirt and connect via a cord to the mold which would fit snugly into one of my ears. This was 1955, and at the time, wearing two big clunky hearing aids at once was considered too cumbersome for a young, active child. I was eleven years old before the development of the much smaller, behind-the-ear power hearing aids, making it possible to wear two aids at once.

Chapter Seven

1. For centuries, the first hearing devices were long ear trumpets. They didn't actually amplify sound but functioned by collecting sound and funneling it down an increasingly narrow tube into the ear. With the Age of Invention and the advent of electricity, all this changed; in 1876 Alexander Graham Bell was awarded a patent for producing a simple receiver that could turn electricity into sound. Then the following year Thomas Edison, who himself had hearing loss, received a patent for inventing a carbon transmitter for the telephone, which amplified the electric signal and increased the overall decibel level by about 15dB. While this volume is not sufficient for most hearing loss, which needs an amplification of at least 30dB, the development of the carbon transmitter resulted in technology that led to carbon hearing aids. These employed a microphone made with a carbon block with cups filled with tiny carbon granules, allowing for currents that amplified the sound to an earpiece.

However, the sound was very scratchy due to the carbon granules, and they also produced a limited frequency range. They were used from 1902 until the 1920s when vacuum tubes were able to increase the amplification up to 70dB. These contraptions, though, were the size of a small bookshelf, and so were totally impractical. By the late 1930s technology improved enough for the development of the first truly wearable hearing aids. These hearing aids had an earpiece (a mold made to fit the outer ear), wire, and receiver worn clipped to the wearer's clothing. The battery pack, however, was large, and had to be strapped to the user's leg.

World War II was a time of tremendous technological innovation, and finally hearing aids were developed with circuit boards and button-sized batteries that allowed all the components to be combined into one unit, about the size of a deck of cards. The units were connected to the earpiece with a thick wire and were the type of hearing aids I had in my early childhood. However, these aids simply amplified the sound evenly across all frequencies, regardless of the level of one's loss at various frequency levels. (The ability to adjust the volume at different frequency levels would come decades later with the advent of digital hearing aids.) And there wasn't yet the ability to put a cap on the amount of volume at a given frequency level, so very loud sounds were extremely painful. That explained why I found very loud noises so distressing. Ironically, extreme loud noises while wearing hearing aids are a real problem for people with severe hearing loss because of the level of amplification required.

Chapter Eight

1. In 1948, Bell Laboratories developed transistors, which led to a major improvement in hearing aids. Transistors replaced the vacuum tubes; they were small, required less battery power, and had less distortion. Eventually these aids were made small enough that two could be worn, one behind each ear. However, digital hearing aids

with microprocessors allowing for audio signals to be separated into different frequency bands that offered fine-tune programming were still decades away.

Chapter Fifteen

1. In 1997 my mother, Marianne Gerhart, was interviewed about her life growing up in Nazi Germany by the United States Holocaust Memorial Museum. The video interview can be accessed online through the following link: https://collections.ushmm.org/search/catalog/irn508410

Acknowledgments

I am grateful to so many friends and family who supported me these past few years in this project. Not only those who directly assisted me in my memoir, but also whose friendship helped hold me and shape who I am now. I couldn't have done it without you.

My first thanks go to Richard Cruwys Brown who acted as midwife to my project. We regularly met over tea in his home to discuss my memoir's initial tender seedlings, which started out as poems.

Then my thanks go to those in my writing group, who encouraged me to write a full-blown memoir. Special mention goes to David Schweidel, our writing teacher, who gave me expert feedback on my early excerpts, and to Barbara Ridley, Gail Kurtz, Alice Feller, and Martina Reaves. And to the others who read and gave me valuable feedback on early chapters and drafts: Andrew Phillips, Jill Ellis, Diana Mei, Susan Ford, Sandra Delay, and Margret Elson.

So many others helped me along the way with their unwavering friendship and belief in me. Special thanks go to Gloria Gregg, who has compassionately listened to my story over almost fifty years of friendship. And thank you to Jane Hausauser, Miriam Eisenhardt, Susan Phillips, Janis Baeuerlen, Helen Brainerd, Abby Pollak, Hilary Lorraine, Julia Partridge, David Firestone, Elizabeth and David Birka-White, Jane Wilson, Dixie Brown, Marianna Goodheart, Roberta Hoffmann, and Suzanne Riess. And to my college buddies who have cheered me on from afar—Margaret Dittemore, Ella Sitkin, Nancy Recasner, and Erica Brotschi. And to Jane Siegel who supported me through a difficult time in my life in London. All of your friendships have so enriched my life.

To my teachers, Hameed Ali and Karen Johnson, of my spiritual path, the Diamond Approach, I hold you with deep gratitude in my heart. Also my love goes out to my fellow travelers—— Beverly Zeien, Diana Clarke, Damaris Moore, Vivienne Kretschemer, Alice Rubenstein, Brian Leahy, Nancy Lovejoy, David Silverstein, Theresa Silow, James Linnehan, Deborah Shappelle, Anne-marie Dietzgen, Jill Davey, Nancy Kirk, Susan Reid, and Batsheva Rotem.

Special thanks go to my friend and piano partner Adrienne Torf for almost ten years of collaborative and joyful music making, and to Donna Seager and Suzanne Gray of the Seager Gray gallery who have believed in me and my painting over so many years.

I am especially grateful to Brooke Warner of She Writes Press who supported me and my memoir from the very beginning. Also, Jodi Fodor, editor extraordinaire; Anne Durette, my copyeditor; Shannon Green, my responsive project manager; Caitlin Hamilton, my publicist; Ashley Shoemaker, my genius marketing guru; and the expert team at She Writes Press who all have made it possible for my memoir to see the light of day.

I extend deep appreciation to my family, who is very dear to me. First, to my parents, I hold an intense gratitude in my heart for passing on to me a profound appreciation of music, art, literature, and beauty which has so enriched my life. My brother Elliot, my nest-mate, provided me great friendship, love, and support over the years, and my stepfather, John Gerhart, showed up for us unfailingly when our father wouldn't. My beloved grandmother, Anna Ernst Zeise, gave me an unconditional love much needed in my childhood. And Monica Gerhart, my sister, Catherine Porter, Elliot's partner, and my nephew Jesse Marseille and his wife Moda Marseille, all bring additional love, support, and joy to my life. I am grateful to my in-laws, Edith and

Farouk Barakat, my sister-in-law Susan Barakat, and Brian Logan, who accepted me wholeheartedly into their family.

Finally, I want to thank my dear daughter Mira Barakat, who gave me the great gift of motherhood. But most importantly, my gratitude goes to my husband, Sam Barakat, for his unwavering support and belief in me, whatever I chose to do. I couldn't have done it without you.

About the Author

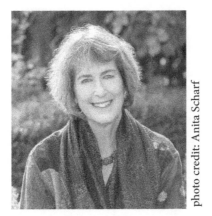

photo credit: Anita Scharf

At age four, Claudia Marseille was diagnosed with a severe hearing loss. With determination and the help of powerful hearing aids, she learned to hear, speak, and lipread. She was mainstreamed in public schools in Berkeley, California. After earning master's degrees in archaeology and public policy, and finally an MFA, she developed a career in photography and painting, a profession compatible with a hearing loss. Claudia ran a fine art portrait photography studio for fifteen years before becoming a full-time painter. Her paintings are represented by the Seager Gray Gallery in Mill Valley, California, and can be seen at www.claudiamarseille.com.

She has played classical piano much of her life. In her free time, she loves to read, watch movies, travel, spend time with friends, and attend concerts and art exhibits. She and her husband live in Oakland and have one grown daughter. Find out more about her memoir at www.claudiamarseilleauthor.com.

Not a Poster Child: Living Well with a Disability—A Memoir by Francine Falk-Allen. $16.95, 978-1631523915
Francine Falk-Allen was only three years old when she contracted polio and temporarily lost the ability to stand and walk. Here, she tells the story of how a toddler learned grown-up lessons too soon; a schoolgirl tried her best to be a "normie," on into young adulthood; and a woman finally found her balance, physically and spiritually.

Loving Lindsey: Raising a Daughter with Special Needs by Linda Atwell. $16.95, 978-1631522802
A mother's memoir about the complicated relationship between herself and her strong-willed daughter, Lindsey—a high-functioning young adult with intellectual disabilities.

Make a Wish for Me: A Family's Recovery from Autism by LeeAndra Chergey. $16.95, 978-1-63152-828-6
A life-changing diagnosis teaches a family that where's there is love there is hope—and that being "normal" is not nearly as important as providing your child with a life full of joy, love, and acceptance.

No Spring Chicken: Stories and Advice from a Wild Handicapper on Aging and Disability by Francine Falk-Allen. $16.95, 978-1-64742-120-5
A companion to Falk-Allen's memoir *Not a Poster Child*, this handbook deftly and humorously shares tips and stories about disability-oriented travel, how to "be with" and adapt to a handicapped or aging person, and simple assistive health care we can employ in order to live our best and longest lives.

Edna's Gift: How My Broken Sister Taught Me to Be Whole by Susan Rudnick. $16.95, 978-1-63152-515-5
When they were young, Susan and Edna, children of Holocaust refugee parents, were inseparable. But as they grew up and Edna's physical and mental challenges altered the ways she could develop, a gulf formed between them. Here, Rudnick shares how her maddening—yet endearing—sister became her greatest life teacher.

Printed in the USA
CPSIA information can be obtained
at www.ICGtesting.com
JSHW021247090524
62837JS00003B/4